PIECE OF ASS

PIECE OF ASS

My Personal Experience With Prostitution in the Ableism Community

Rollon Rebel

with Cedric Quincy

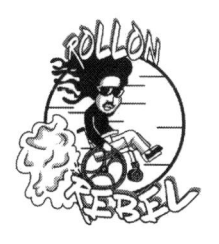

WWW.ROLLONREBEL.COM

Saint Louis ■ Atlanta

Rollon Rebel titles are published by
Rollon Rebel, LLC., 7253 Watson Road PMB 1303, Saint Louis, Missouri 63119

Book Credits

Authors: Tony "Rollon Rebel" and Cedric Quincy
Models: Rollon Rebel
Cover Photographer: Vanick
Cover Designer: Emmanuel D. Simms
Interior Layout: Cedric Quincy for Write Sing Work, LLC
Editors: Bethany Hamilton Freebird

First Rollon Rebel Publication August 2024

10 9 8 7 6 5 4 3 2 1

PIECE OF ASS
Copyright ©2024 Derrick Sykes

ISBN: 979-8-9852912-2-3 (eBook)
ISBN: 979-8-9852912-3-0 (print)

This book is a sexual memoir of the subject Tony Rebel. The publisher acknowledges these are his recollections of the events that have have taken place and all others are not held liable for the information contained herein in this or previous versions oh the book. Some names and identifying characteristics have been changed to protect the privacy of the individuals involved.

No part of this work may be reproduced or copied in any form or by any means— graphic, electronic, or mechanical, including photocopying, taping or information storage and retrieval system—without the written consent of Rollon Rebel, LLC

Printed in the United States of America & Canada

CONTENTS

Introduction: Pressure	9
Let's Talk About Sex	14
Hollywood Dreams	22
Gay 4 Pay	30
I Endorse These Strippers	39
Touch My Body	54
Magic Stick	63
Sex & Candy	69
Sex Room	74
Me, Myself and I	82
Pills N Potions	91
Thinking With My Dick	99
Full Disclosure	104
Aye Papi	116
Doin' It	128
Too Tough	136
The Apprentice	146

Pound Cake	150
Militant	156
SupHomie	168
Someday Is Tonight	177
Afterword	184
Works Cited	188
Acknowledgments	189
About the Authors	191

WARNING

This book contains descriptions of high-risk sexual activity including unprotected sex, random hook ups, and paying for sexual services. While the Rollon Rebel's recollections of these encounters are personal in nature, it is not recommended for the readers or the general community to participate in these activities.

There is a danger to soliciting or being solicited for paid sexual encounters including but not limited to:
* theft
* assault
* kidnapping
* trafficking
* transmission of sexual and contact diseases
* high risk for body mutilation
* high risk for being maimed
* high risk of death

IT IS NOT RECOMMENDED BY THE AUTHORS, PUBLISHER, OR ANY ENTITY INVOLVED IN THE PRODUCTION OR DISTRIBUTION OF THIS BOOK THAT ANY OF THE ACTIVITIES BE RECREATED IN ANY FORM.

We do not assume any responsibility for any encounters you may have with individuals mentioned or implied in this book.

Play safe, wrap up, get tested.

AUTHOR'S NOTE

Derrick Sykes, known to most people as Tony "Rollon" Rebel has been writing and dictating this book with Cedric Quincy since June 2017. While it is the intention to create a factual book, certain names, descriptions, locations and/or events were altered and changed to protect the privacy of certain individuals and organizations. The recollections in this story are Tony's version of the events that have taken place.

DEDICATION

I dedicate this book to everyone in the disabled community that may feel like they don't have a voice you can do it. I know some of the subjects are a bit taboo but here we are. Some of you may be uncomfortable, However, I am sorry in advance. My mission is to shed light to a topic that is not talked about. Like the principles of my beloved Sigma, Social Action and Education is the goal. I dedicate this book to my frat brothers, mentors friends and family that have supported my throughout this journey. Most importantly I dedicate this to my mother because I know it has been hard raising a disabled son and I know you worry about me. I want you to know that the pride determination and life lessons that you have taught me have not gone unnoticed. It is because of you I am who I am today and I want to say thank and I hope I make you proud.

Love,

Your Son

PART ONE - EXPLANATION

INTRODUCTION: PRESSURE

Prostitution is considered one of the oldest professions in the world. Traditionally dominated by women, usually unmarried and assumed to have had to fend for themselves because they were single. When I was in school, my teacher taught me that history books referred to prostitutes as being an "actress."

"What other job would a woman have in which they would have gotten paid for their work?"

Sit and think about it–wives of some of the "greatest" men in history: Constantine, Justenian, Mark Anthony, were indeed, prostitutes. It makes perfect sense if they were "making their own money" without the support of a man. In Biblical times, women had to marry men or be in the care of their father in order to keep and sustain wealth. There are not many references in history that the majority acknowledge that show how women got and sustained wealth outside of sex at first.

Whether that is by design or by sexism is not for debate at the moment, nor is it the subject of this book. We have gathered here to talk about how money or favors are exchanged for lucid sexual encounters only meant to be satisfying to one party.

Men have prostituted but have not been celebrated in the way women have. They've been employed to keep rich women company and to discreetly supply companionship to powerful men. Perhaps some of it was to hide their own sexual satisfaction but that's not something known either.

Our society has frowned upon the practice due to "religious" and "moral standards." It's considered "the easy way out." I would disagree—prostitutes provide a service that should be sought out legally and taxed. There are many who feel that sexual crimes would decrease if prostitution and the use of their services weren't stigmatized. There should be regulations such as mandatory testing and full disclosures of statuses. Protection and safety measures to make sure the women and men who provide the service are taken care of. I'm for HIV and full STI panel testing of every sex worker in the streets and on camera. There should be some sort of registration so that there is no question whether a worker is legit and of legal age. I wouldn't go as far as to say maintain a license, like I do when I practice therapy and mental health services but, something should be done.

In the same breath I say that, I acknowledge that with the same energy we are taking care of the prostitutes and other adult entertainers—we need to make sure the Johns are treated with respect. Without the men and women who pay for sexual services and companionship, there wouldn't be a profession. Just like Johns shouldn't be verbally and physically abusive toward the prostitute—the John should be treated with dignity and respect.

The prostitute may provide the service but the John has to be willing to pay.

Let Hollywood tell it, it's only "the ugly ass dudes" who acquire the services. Some bald-headed fat motherfucker, with beady-eyes, missing teeth and stank breath. Wet stringy hair with sweat fighting to escape, dripping on his clothes. Reeking of smoke and rank man scent, he's begging and pleading with some pretty bitch to put her mouth on his stank, Vienna sausage-sized penis that he can barely grip in his hand. One she knows she's going to barely feel inside of her once he mounts and she's gotta fake pleasure from every pump he makes and every bead of sweat that lands on her chest. That's what they show us on television, which helps propel the stereotype that prostitution is not a needed service.

Everyone overlooks the lonely people, who don't necessarily want sex but a human being in their presence they can talk to. Or the "rich person" who just wants a date for the night.

What many people don't understand is that those of us on the ableism spectrum are frequent patrons of professional sexual services. When I say ableism, for the purposes of this book, I'm covering a broad range of mental and physical disabilities. From what you "think" you can see, to those who are able to keep their disabilities a secret. Those of us on the ableism spectrum who participate in prostitution go from paying for companionship to wanting to be voyeurs to full on sexual encounters. Oftentimes, we pay a high cost because we are deemed to be "difficult" to deal with. Truth is, "difficult" may mean unattractive to the person providing the services. I know of some instances where other Johns have been asked to wear a face mask or a pillowcase when receiving the service or to wear a costume to hide the "disability" so that the service can be rendered correctly. Fucked up that we often have to accommodate the performer who is being paid to make sure one of our physiological hierarchy of needs is being met. Ironically, we are often taken advantage of once the prostitute finds out we are the John. It's not uncommon for prostitutes to have us pay for services we don't receive or we are brutalized and robbed all for just wanting a human interaction.

    I know the feeling because I've been a victim of several assaults and scams from some of your favorite prostitutes, escorts and porn stars. Because I'm not afraid to use my voice to speak up on these issues and to call these assholes out for their blatant disrespect and ridicule, I'm an outcast. I'm called every name but a child of God, meanwhile, I have video evidence and a paper trail of some of these incidents occurring. It's a damn if I do, damn it I don't scenario. When I'm silent and say nothing, I watch motherfuckers get implants or go on expensive trips with money they stole from me.

The physical scars they leave may heal but the mental and emotional abuse they inflict me with still lingers. Even with this, I still can't stay away. I need sex and relationships are not easy to get into.

Some would say I have an addiction.

Maybe that's true, but I think there's more to this. It's the longing and desire to be treated like a human being. The right to experience intimacy–not be alone. I feel that I, and others in my position, deserve companionship. It's rare that I see romantic love involving a person in the ableism community–I've only briefly experienced it here and there. Even with that, there is a level of guilt because I know that while I have, many don't ever experience it at all.

Ultimately, the reason I'm writing this book is for respect. For myself as a person, yes, but for those of us most deserving of love, yet least likely to truly experience it.

LET'S TALK ABOUT SEX

I am writing *Piece of Ass* because I want to talk about sex. S-E-X. I don't just want to recite the lyrics to the Salt N Pepa hit that took them to the top of the Billboard Charts in 1993.

I want to talk about sex—not just the physical act of penetration—but the intimacy, relationships, love and lust that are built on this act. Whether it's in a committed relationship, a regular hook up with a trusted partner, or a random "off the wall" encounter from cruising, I want to talk about it.

No one wants to believe that I am having sex—which is insulting to say the least.

Just because I am in this wheelchair due to my cerebral palsy diagnosis, doesn't mean that I am incapable of human emotions. People feel that it is okay to talk about my sexual desires and needs without including me in the conversation. They act like I'm supposed to be discussed and argued about—decisions made for me without my input.

Well fuck that—and if you support that line of thinking, well, fuck you, too.

I, Derrick A. Sykes, known to you as Tony Rollon Rebel, am capable of speaking for myself and advocating for those with needs similar to mine who can't speak up for themselves.

I'm guilty of being confrontational—that's the story my adversaries sell when they get on Instagram and Facebook Live and these YouTube reality shows. It's what makes them important. They get on social media and Beyonce's internet to spread lies and to gossip about what they *think* I'm doing. Meanwhile, when I'm not counseling a person learning to accept their HIV status, I'm helping a family understand the nuances of having a child on the LGBTQ spectrum.

In my previous book, one of my major goals was to be able to tell *my story*. Not being screamed at by some deranged lunatic. Not to experience the constant harassment and threats to my life

For three years before we put pen to pad (or we dictated over forty hours worth of recordings and numerous conversations before, during and after), we set out to determine what my story would be. We wanted to talk about what it's like being in a wheelchair, having to advocate for myself and just some of the incidents I've been in.

As we were putting this story together, some things were shared by my nemesis that I didn't have a chance to address. My nudes were leaked and I was ridiculed for how I looked naked. I was the talk of the social media circles I was a part of. I can't change how I look—you like it or you don't.

They said this shit like I'm supposed to be ashamed that I had the audacity to take a picture of myself sprawled on top of the bed like I'm a fucking supermodel.

I am, bitch!

Like I'm supposed to be ashamed of being naked in my own home.

I'm not.

I wish I had taken control over how my nudes (cause I got more than those) were shared but we're here. Yes, I laid across the crisp white linen sheets spread across the bed and showed my backside. All of my perfections and imperfections to see, share and be ridiculed.

I did it—let's move on.

And before I talk more sex stuff—my audition tape for a reality show. I guess a bitch was wrong for not getting glammed up for you niggas–but I don't live in a world of make believe. I'm not one of the *Real Housewives of Atlanta*, married to the right nigga or bringing in the right amount of cash to keep an assistant around to keep me beat for the gods. I'm a motherfuckin' human being that has a disability that keeps me from controlling my bodily functions, at times. I need help with basic house care duties sometimes because guess what? I can't get *everywhere* in this fuckin' chair. I wish you people, you motherfuckin' people who talk about me all gotdamn day could trade places with me for a moment. Experience my despair, my trauma, living life without the advantages of being pretty. Understand what Tionne was saying in her Grammy nominated song.

Next, stories came out about some of the men I have allegedly had encounters with. Some aren't true and I'll get to clarifying those stories momentarily. Others, who were paid handsomely to bring me a few moments of pleasure have flat out denied the encounters took place.

Or lied about what took place in order to shame me for profits or to modify their own pathetic lives.

Which is unfortunate because I literally have receipts from my credit cards to the PayPal, Ca$hApp, Zelle accounts and other preferred payment processors I used to pay for these services. I've subscribed to OnlyFans accounts and tipped these motherfuckers just to entertain me and then what? I've paid some of these men hundreds—thousands of dollars over the years. And I will talk about that too, since y'all brought it up.

When I told Cedric, I wanted to write a book, I initially set out to do one memoir detailing my story and experiences. I was going to include many of my scandalous tales in what I'd set out to be my magnum opus. *Don't Get*

F+cked Up was initially called *Hopelessly Bound*. The cover had depicted a vision of me breaking the chains I felt bound by—my wheelchair in the center of the madness. At the start of producing this book, my life was on a different path. I initially wrote a draft of the book by myself and due to some unforeseen circumstances, lost it and was unable to recover it or the initial Facebook account I had where I had shared the book with a couple of people.

As we set out to revise *Don't Get F+cked Up*, we understood that my sexcapades needed their own book. I paid for enough encounters to last a few books really—but I don't just want to talk about the men I've had sex with. This isn't meant to be a kiss and tell kind of book. I want to educate people on the physical and mental psychology that comes with people with special needs manifesting and engaging in sexual encounters. When I talk with others who have diagnoses similar to mine—or who can function with their diagnoses to the level that I can, I found that many of us share a similar story. We go the extra mile to get glammed up to the gods to appear attractive. Make our chairs, walkers and other equipment we used to function disappear. We bring our human form to the table—but most importantly, we present our hearts as sacrifices in order to experience the kind of love and passion that comes with being intimate.

Or in lust.

Or to pay to satisfy our lusts.

Cedric was telling me about a known mental and physical health advocate who admitted publicly that they paid for sex. We won't reveal their identity here and going forward, we will discuss them and others whom we may reference using they/them pronouns. I wasn't as shocked by the revelation as he appeared to be because being the John for all these escorts was the story of my life. I was shocked that they admitted this aloud and that this admission was caught on film. And while their admission wasn't the main point of their discussion—it was one that had an impact on me.

Being a John and being a special needs person who pays a premium for this need to be met should be discussed more frequently. I know I can't speak for all, but the truth is participating in prostitution is how many of us get it in. Paying sex workers for satisfaction was like our dirty little secret and we were shamed. I'm blessed that I have a job and as I continue to get education and fight for the right to employment and independence, I can continue to satisfy my needs. To some extent, this has been an advantage because my money has made it possible for me to pay for men whom many consider to be out of my league. On the contrary, one of the scariest things I've learned is that I could have almost any man I want for the *right* price.

Yet, no one considers the price *I pay* for these encounters. It's more than the money I've paid. The arguments I've gotten into with the escorts and other personalities are petty at best. The shade we throw each other helps others stay relevant and enhance their platforms. I don't benefit from these transactions—at best they bruise my ego but at their worst, they're part of the reason there is an unjust negative perception of me. Usually, those instances are my best-case scenario. I have been scammed by quite a few of your favorite adult entertainers, independent musicians and escorts. A few have physically or sexually assaulted me (a nod to the warning labels that appear on both books). There are at least two, violent robberies where more than my pride was injured. I've ruined a few friendships and burnt some bridges professionally and personally. I've begged and pleaded with quite a few of these individuals to do right by me—stop lying on me—and now we've reached an impasse.

I'm not here to hurt anyone's feelings, or make anyone believe me. But I will not be denied my right to tell my truth. It's not always pretty. I've had to hold myself accountable for my actions. But most of all, I've had to be willing to share parts of myself I wanted to deny existed.

I cannot be a licensed professional mental health counselor if I cannot be real with myself. In my work, I deal with people who discover and deal with their HIV status, other sexual assault victims and those who are dealing with LGBTQ issues.

I am so tired of you motherfuckers questioning me about how this looks as a therapist. I know some may look at this as an addiction, which it is, but also it is my liberation. It's also buying love as you say, but guess what? When you cooking and cleaning for that no good dude that beat yo ass, is that an addiction or buying love? When he cheats on you with other men or women is that love? Or having multiple girlfriends or boyfriends but you're not the main but you take them back. My title has nothing to do with my reality. This is temporary. Some things did not happen the way I wanted but I will not give up. I want my forever partner but until I get him I am going to show imperfect but ready and willing. You bitches love calling out flaws. Yes, I am a therapist that has dealt with escorts but I am honest because the person on my couch could commit suicide because of shame. You hoes are dumb, this message is bigger than me. I do not want peopl to live bound by my trauma like I did. So if you are judging me because you don't like me, the message is simple. Judge yo mammy and her choice to swallow you

Sex is a large part of my life—not just the physical act. But I want to talk about that—let's go.

HOLLYWOOD DREAMS

Growing up, every movie or television show I saw went like this:

Boy meets girl

Boy married girl

Boy and girl life happily ever after

I'm not gonna lie, I fell for the idealism that one day, I'd find a man who'd want to live happily ever after with me. I knew I was gay and would substitute "woman" with "man" since they didn't have that representation available for me. In the vision that was serviced to me, I didn't see men paying women or other men for sexual favors. I didn't see those of us with mental or physical disabilities because to most people, we didn't exist.

We were the people everyone hid in their closets or their basements and only brought out at family gatherings. Our meals were out on trays and delivered to us twice a day.

When people saw us, it was a rare outing because we really weren't supposed to be seen or heard.

History used to teach us that the first time people with mental or physical disabilities were able to make their presence known were in circuses and "side-shows." If you look at the vintage flyers for them or the state fairs, they always promoted someone with a physical disability as a "freak." Every now and then we were included with the picture but most of the time we either were a byline, or a caption listed next to the other people who are considered freaks. And animals, we were equated to animals. We were placed in chains or cages and put on display for all to see. We were exploited for other peoples financial gain because we looked different. No one cared that we were people with feelings, or emotions, which is part of the problem with people not seeing us as sexual beings now. All people cared about was the ability of being able to see us one time, just so they'd have something to talk about for their Sunday dinner.

Fuck those people and fuck you, too, if you feel like this is the only form of representation we should be allowed to have. We are human beings and being a sexual being part of being a human being. We deserve to be part of the conversation and we deserve to have sex for free just like everybody else.

I think the first time I saw a physically disabled person would be the short black men—Emmanuel Webster and Gary Coleman in reruns of *Webster* and *Different Strokes*.

These were young men when they were first introduced to us and regardless of what they've accomplished after the cancelation of their shows, the world continued to see them as children, not adults. The shows lasted as long as they were able to be kids and once they were grown, the shows disappeared. Rarely did we see them show interest in love of either sex. I don't remember hearing anyone say they were attractive. These two men were described with antidotes of "cute", "adorable", "lovable" and other traits that could apply equally to kids and pets. To be completely honest, I believe most people would rather the young men be pets. When the actors ran into the problems in "real life", I noticed how people and the tabloids focused on their child-like qualities.

A few characters that were blind or hearing impaired were treated like props. On rare occasions, they'd be talked about in conversations, have voice overs or acknowledged in some form. Once they made an appearance and their disability was revealed, it was treated like "oh, *that's why* I never saw them" and then they were removed.

The first movie I saw with a person with physical disabilities displayed front and center was *Forrest Gump*. The lead character, played by Tom Hanks, had a crooked spine that forced him to wear leg braces, according to Wikipedia and other sources. His friend, Bubba, who was black, was said to be on the autism spectrum. The love interest, Jenny, continuously chose other men over him, except for that one time she gave him some. And that's what I had to look forward to. I didn't deserve love or sex because someone wanted to be active with me–in the back of my mind, I felt like if it was done, it was from sympathy that I wasn't able-bodied enough to receive it on my own. In some ways, I felt like the movie reinforced that we weren't deserving of love and affection.

I'm not blaming the movie for the situation I'm in now. I do acknowledge that some of my need to pay content creators for sex comes from low self-esteem. I think this is the first time I've admitted out loud that I don't always find myself attractive. I have sex with people to convince myself I can bring value to people's lives and I'm willing to pay for sex to prove to myself that anyone is obtainable. There's a part of me that becomes attached once I pay for and receive the service, but it fulfills the human connection that I need. And I think as men, especially black men, we're not given the freedom to talk about our social-emotional issues surrounding sex much. We're not able to talk about it amongst our friends, our peers, or any other associations we belong in. We're expected to present the macho-man persona that has sex a lot, full of testosterone and the ability to satisfy anyone we give our dicks to.

The first time many of us hear we are handsome and validated for our looks is from our mamas. A part of me thinks that the root of the emotional incest so many black men have with our mothers, but that's not to topic of this book. I can count on one hand and not use all my fingers how many times a woman has told me they thought I was handsome.

Deep down, it's been my experience that many black men often don't hear that they are physically or sexually attractive unless they fit certain criteria. We have to have the perfect facial features, Athletically, athletic defined body, have the perfect swagger, or presentation. Once we cross that hurdle, we have to have a certain level of intelligence, make a certain amount of money, work a "six figure job", and have certain material possessions to be deemed worthy of dating. Thanks to social media, I know now that I'm not to take any woman, or any man to any well-known "fine dining establishment. Oh yeah, and I almost forgot, I need to be "10 inches or bigger," according to Left Eye of TLC.

Nowhere in the description I gave above does having a physical or mental disability that anyone's description of a perfect mate. It's not even acceptable to be a "friend with benefits" or regular "fuck buddy." Who wants to brag that they're creeping with or having casual sex with someone who doesn't appear to be normal. I get it—there are some that view a casual sexual relationship with a person with disabilities as that person being taken advantage of.

What if that's what I want? Wait—not all the time or literally. But what if I were in a casual sexual relationship that didn't involve money?

As time passed, I've started to see a few more representations, but the truth is, I can't name a well-known black man with a noticeable physical impairment. I'm sure there are some that are known locally, and this is not meant to define someone's celebrity or status. But let's be honest, name a single man that is a sex symbol that has a noticeable limb missing or other deformity.

I'll wait.

Oh, you get my point. We don't exist. That's one of the main points of writing this book. Pointing out that in any case, we're good enough as long as someone can get a check off of our disability, but often we're left out of the conversation when it comes to being partners. We're not even thought of. We're a special class, one that usually has to have certain boxes to fit into this class. Then we're worth something to someone. That's how I've been made to feel. That's the part for many people when they get into conversations with people who may have similar disabilities that I can't truly relate to.

They care to emphasize with me.

I'm not saying that all people with mental or physical disabilities have to pay for sex. I think our abilities to be seen as sexual beings would be better if we were presented that way without being exploited. Which leaves me to the elephant in the room. One place where those of us with physical or mental disabilities have a representation is adult entertainment. This is our new circus. We're regulated to a special category in which we're promoted for either being "little people," in wheelchairs," or for being "freaks."

Yup, we're back at the goddamn circus. Always hope that one day we get to leave. Doesn't seem like it's gonna happen anytime soon. And before anyone accuses me of throwing shade, I'm aware of certain "celebrities" and I use that term very loosely, who happened to be physically disabled. Some are even in wheelchairs like me. But what are we famous for really? Our disability comes in the question when we're always accused of scamming, fighting, or misrepresenting being black and being disabled. For those whom I won't mention, we're not even being given the decency of being imperfect, which is another human character trait we're deprived of. But we are an embarrassment, and that's the place. A lot of people would prefer us to be.

I'd like to have my own *Moonlight* story one day. I'd like to see a television show or identify with a main character who was basically impaired, and gay. Have relationships with another human being, I'm even open to different identities. It would be nice to have our own *Posse* or Noah's Arc. I like my own Wade, Praytell, or Lil' Murda. We could fit any role if we were given that opportunity. It would be nice if we were given the chance to show off our bodies pleasantly and be praised for having traits that are physically fit counterparts are blessed to have.

It would be nice to even have a porn star that would be able to transcend our category and have sex with mainstream performers. I don't know where one's gonna come from and I realize it could probably take a few more decades before we get to this point. Perhaps put out there, the universal bless us , ready to step into the role by the next generation of age.

I don't know if that's my Hollywood dream, but I think that would be a good place to start.

GAY 4 PAY

"I see you got my money," Lamar smiled.

The arrangement of fifty and twenty dollar bills were placed on the table as I looked myself over in my chair. I was in my blue and white FUBU sweatsuit at the time. As I looked into the mirror of the Sleep Inn I'd rented for the night, I could see my freshly cut taper fade making me look "so fresh and so clean" as Outkast would say. The Curve cologne I wore was subtle, but not overwhelming.

This contrasted with the Polo cologne that permeated from Lamar's six foot one, one hundred and ninety pound frame. His stone cold face with sharp features would've made him a perfect fit for the hard-looking, "hood nigga" image that Taggaz and DawgPoundUSA were going for. He had on an Allen Iverson jersey and some loose-fitting Tommy Hilfiger jeans—a sharp contrast from the white wife beater and the baggy jeans I was used to him wearing.

His Air-Force Ones stayed crisp, however.

In our dealings with each other, he kept his athletic frame intact and thanks to his multiple trips to the gym, his muscles became more pronounced over time. I wouldn't say he turned into GI Joe but if Sterling K. Brown ever needed a body double, at that point in time, Lamar could fit the bill.

Unlike my first encounter where he rammed his cut nine and a half inch Snickers bar into my mouth, I was going to feel this meat in my hole. Lamar was gentle when he unsnapped the straps and braces that helped keep me in my chair. Before I'd had the chance to enjoy being lifted in the air, I was roughly tossed on the queen size bed like a rag doll. I could tell the hotel had just gotten new mattresses from the way I bounced up a few inches and multiple times. This bed was firm and hard like a trampoline.

Once again, I had no control as my sweat clothes were snatched off of me and I was butt naked, positioned in the doggystyle position, facing the headboard.

I wanted to look in the mirror. I thought as I could feel the slightly cool liquid gel from the personal lubricant moisturizing my asshole. I was fortunate to have crouched in the right position and locked in my elbows because not even a second after feeling the lubricant, I felt most of Lamar inside of me. I was somewhat shocked and surprised, but I should have known better because while Lamar had a soft, sensitive side when we talked–Lamar liked it rough when we fucked.

He grinded his hips on my ass, his pubic hairs brushing my ass crack. His balls were long enough to slap mine with each stroke. As I was being worked on my backside, I'd struggle to catch my breath. Lamar had placed his socked foot on the side of my head and it was strong enough to keep me down. My moans and groans might've suggested that I was in ecstasy, my body knew I wasn't in pleasure.

I was paying one hundred dollars for Lamar to ram his dick into me and he was giving me a rushed performance. It was pissing me off because I was wise enough to schedule this appointment at least four hours before he had to get ready for another ballroom performance. He had won the last competition he had wearing the Allen Iverson jersey that was now crumpled up on the floor and with a realistic looking man-unit that incorporated the professional basketball player's signature zig-zag cornrows. If you didn't know him outside of the ball, you would've never known that he had a tight fade under the man-unit and that his waves made a permanent ripple on top of his head.

The latex from the condom he wore burned with each stroke. I tried to lift my head up but I understood first hand what it felt like to have a man have his foot on your neck.

"I need—" I struggled to breathe and could feel my chest move up and down with each stroke I was given. "Lube. LUBE!" I tried to yell but I was being drowned out from all the "bitch niggas" and "faggots" he was calling me. And that's another thing I wasn't liking about these encounters, Lamar felt the need to degrade me as if he didn't need my money as bad as I needed his dick. He was on his second bottle of cologne that I bought. The Air-Force Ones were replacements from the pair he got last month because that pair had too many creases in it. I didn't know at the time what he was wearing for his competition that night but I'm sure between the head I paid for two days ago and the last session, where he barely lasted three or four minutes, paid for that.

Don't get me wrong, I loved watching Lamar perform and I got a kick over how the average person wouldn't know he was gay. The roughneck image looked good on Lamar and I loved watching him flex on other people and how he made them his bitch. Kind of turned me on. When people saw us in public, many thought he was my caretaker and I learned to play along with it because it made our sex better.

Lamar growled like a damn bear when he came and without warning, I could feel air rush into my hole when he pulled out. I also thought I felt a little blood because I never got the lube I was requesting. My hole felt like it was in tune with my heartbeat–throbbing and sore.

"You coming to the ball tonight?" He asked as I was barely able to turn myself over. Just like that, my masculine, thug escort turned into an excited child who was nervous about his first performance. I liked it rough but my hole was tapping out–wanting to surrender from the experience.

"It's at eight o'clock, right?" I brought the sheets up to cover my nude body. Lamar was rushing to brush his teeth and rinse his mouth while he brushed his fade.

"Yeah," he confirmed as he sprayed another layer of Polo on his pulse points and on his clothes.

"Why don't you take a shower here and then go over there and get dressed?" I offered. I hated to see him rush from our encounter because it made me feel like he was repulsed to be in my presence.

Lamar was athletic, attractive to many and kept an extensive clientele—I hated to be reminded of that. I knew as a John, my place was to be served, to pay and to keep it moving but in this stage of my development with escorts, I hadn't grasped the concept of having the next man on deck. It wasn't as easy as it appeared. Ideally, I'd get the room—as I'd done this night, let Lamar do his thing—and it still makes my hole twitch as I retell this—*and have the next nigga lined up.* That's the part I'd miss, having the next man lined up. I would later experience that but I wanted the "boyfriend experience." I needed to get to a point where I was paying these guys to spend the night. I hated the idea that I was paying to begin with because I couldn't believe that Lamar was not enjoying himself. We spent too much time outside of this for it not to be that. I knew he had to prepare for a ball after he got his nut off but I can't help how I feel. It's not about being a bitch but longing to have someone I could call my own. I longed for the days where I wasn't paying Lamar for dick but as long as he had men from St. Louis to Cali to Tokyo and Dubai demanding his services, I'd have to learn how to be the best client so I'd get the most out of this time.

I didn't go to the balls just to see Lamar, I was actually surprised with the variety of different men I'd find at the balls. A ball was a competition between different groups of men and women who belonged to different "houses." A house is an association of men and possibly women who have a fraternity-like connection that bonds them to different members within the house. A lot of the competitions I've seen have different themes and the categories promote looking and acting like the theme. The participants compete for prizes and bragging rights.

St. Louis did not have a huge ballroom scene on the scale of what could be seen in New York, Atlanta or Los Angeles. I will say the guys and gals out here had heart and people traveled hundreds of miles to participate in our events. It was at the balls that I found out that Lamar made almost a quarter of a million a year for the past few years between all of his clients. He made more money than most black men in corporate America. Had me wondering why I went to college to begin with. The ballroom brought different types of men: corporate, flamboyant, athletic, college, blue collar, fraternity men and no matter what their position was in life, they all wanted to be entertained and they all had money to spend.

Going to the balls allowed me to forget that I had cerebral palsy. Forced me to make sure my presence was on point at all times–I couldn't afford to be caught slipping. My personal appearance became everything as I used it to measure my self-esteem. My Karl Kani looked better than yours. I had the latest designer before you even thought of it. I worked hard and I made sure I competed harder.

Lamar was my first introduction into escorting and prostitution and over the years, I made a vow to find a man who would love me for me. One I didn't have to pay for companionship—one that would bring mutual benefits. I'd have a few boyfriends. Some were good—most were horrible encounters. Lamar would introduce me to a few men, who inadvertently became my tricks as well. Some of the men were within his own house and others he competed with. Some of the men only wanted me as a client so they could compete with Lamar and fuck with him.

Lamar would also introduce me to a few people who would go on to become adult entertainers and shape some of the experiences I've dealt with in this book. I wouldn't say he created a monster or stirred my addiction but I will say having sex with "gay celebrities" has come with a set of headaches and heartaches I wouldn't wish on no one. It's brought some drama and chaos I wouldn't have expected to happen. One minute, I'm some lusting John who has to pay for sex so I can experience intimacy. Next minute, I'm being tricked out of my professional services under the guise of "friendship" and "love lost".

While I don't blame him, Lamar created an unequal power vacuum that I've never been able to reset. One that sees me as a member of a lower caste in society even though I'm the one that has to have the money, the place to host the encounter, and do the bulk of the legwork to insure the encounter happens. I take the risk—I pay the deposit for services that aren't provided, I pay in full to have some of your faves not be able to get hard (don't worry motherfuckers, I treat y'all better than y'all have ever treated me because Cedric won't let me put y'all names in this book YOU'RE WELCOME!!!), I pay for half-assed or lackluster performance. Found out that all performances we saw on some of our favorite porn clips or on those fan pages weren't real.

When I accepted life as a gay black man, I'd never thought I'd live in a world where the people who are shunned and outcast in regular society are the rockstars here. Bobby Blake, Tiger Tyson, Jovonnie, Castro, Phat Daddy became our Michael Jordan, Shannon Sharpe, Tiger Woods, Venus & Serena Williams. Our porn stars are the perfect C-List celebrities because we know more about them than some of the actual celebrities, politicians and local people who have actual influence in our lives. We don't just beat our meats and fantasize about them while we stick PhatRabbitKiller's dildo in our asses. Our porn stars were always accessible to us—even before the days of social media, we could find some of our faves in our own neighborhoods if we lived in New York, Philly, Charlotte or Atlanta. A few of them (who I will also not name) live or are from in St. Louis, too. Before social media, these men were in the ballroom (a few belong to houses), upscale gay parties and worked for other well-known celebrities who were not aware of their "gay activities." In the black gay community, we know more about these men (and women) than we know about our own family members.

And I get it. In the black gay community, escorting has been how we've provided a life for each other. Some have built wealth with it but most have been able to change any and everything physically and mentally. Men who have chosen or want to identify with become women or whatever they want to call themselves. Built our own communities and have provided our own support networks. We've become family and regardless of our roles in it, we all need each other. Without them, I can't get no dick (and we won't talk about what I have to go through to get some ass) and without me, they can't get paid.

Welcome to the toxic relationship.

I ENDORSE THESE STRIPPERS

$50 to suck his dick.

For those of y'all who read *Don't Get F+cked Up*, I told the story of how I wasn't searching for Lamar to become his John. In some ways, I was coerced and tricked into this sexual encounter. Being forced to pay for sex. I thought Lamar and I were better than that and I added this trauma and mental stress to what I'd already suppressed being a rape victim. I never understood or addressed how I was good enough to be forced to perform a sexual act but not enough to give consent without having to pay for it.

Ain't that shit backwards—I should be getting sex for free.

Never mind. Don't let me give these simple-minded, self-entitled pretty privileged pricks something else to bitch about.

As I paid Lamar and later his gay sisters Deiondre and Vonte, I found my self-esteem being chipped away. I questioned whether I was ugly—I'd heard it all my life but what about my features that I couldn't control made me so undesirable? If I were meant to be an invalid, why did I get born with sexual desires and preferences? Why couldn't I have been a eunuch? I think I love touching my dick and playing with it as much as the next man. Why did I discover pleasure from the male G-spot the way I did if I was going to have so much problems getting there?

Then, if self-doubt weren't enough, I wondered how much this new expense was going to cost me and how often was I going to have to pay for it? Couldn't I get these niggas on a coupon or something? I felt degraded knowing that I couldn't just consensually put my mouth on someone's penis without a price. But in my first sexual encounter, it was done to me.

It's not ironic—it's disgraceful.

I sucked it up, pun intended, and like a good escort, Lamar promoted that I was a new John willing to support the girls. Even though Lamar wanted me exclusively to be his client, I learned that he'd have no loyalty to me, because I wasn't the only one paying him for his services. Lamar was fucking niggas that I wouldn't have blinked at yet had the nerve to judge me because I sat in this chair and at times couldn't control all of my bodily functions. When Lamar was at the top of his game, Lamar would have been an actor's equivalent to say Will Smith or Tom Cruise. In all the right action movies—hard enough to win the fights but sensual enough to prove that he could lay it down in the bedroom. The random peaks at his cheeks through his sagging jeans reminded me of the artwork for the original James Earl I Hardy novels. When I was around him, I was the gay boy who wore street clothes to fit in with the down low/DL thug image.

It was through him that I met and got entangled deeper into the ballroom world. I perfected my attraction to rugged, masculine-presenting, light skin men. There, I admit it, that was my preference. Not the "so light you thought they were white" boys. Some of the ones I was attracted to would fail a paper bag test. In the ballroom, these were the guys I encouraged to win. I love the way they were underestimated and assumed to be feminine because of their complexion. In some ways, I saw these men as the opposite as me as they moved fluidly while I was confined. Let them tell it the men had the pick of the litter and I was lucky if they took a shit on me.

Overcoming the mental abuse that comes with this relationship is not a challenge I welcome to face head on. I bury it in my work—I do my best to help others see the best in themselves and be able to be a confidant as they solve their problems. When my therapy clients achieve their goals and dreams, I feel like I've defeated my own demons. I want to jump up and cheer for them, yet when I forget my position and try I'm desperately reminded I can't. At that moment I pray that my clients remember the clarity I've provided for their mind and not the inability to physically control my body.

While I appreciate that my physical condition hasn't prevented me from doing my job, I hate how I'm judged outside of that. Seen as less than human. The hardest part about being physically handicapped is the way people try to take advantage of you. It's like people have no good intentions with me. There's an automatic perception of weakness because I can't stand up to you and look you in the eye. I have to roll fast, not walk, not run if I'm trying to get away from someone. Because of my chair, I often have to face issues head-on. My legs aren't strong, but that doesn't mean I can't get in a good punch. I've always had good upper body dexterity. The lack of strength in my legs doesn't mean I can't throw dick, I just don't always get the opportunity to do so.

Where a lot of content creators fuck up is they try to be someone online that they're not. To be honest a lot of them don't want to be sex workers. They want to be regular people with respectable jobs and healthy careers. Many of these guys have masters degrees and work two or three part-time jobs just to make ends meet. Some are guys who just picked up a camera and got lucky they did the right scene, with the right partner. Because that didn't work out and they want easy fast money and they know men will pay for graphic, "exclusive" content, they think they have an easy path in. I get that. I've been there where after I got my degrees, went through hell to get my therapists licenses in two states and struggled living on disability, the money still isn't good. It's like, "what the fuck did I go to school for of all I had to do to be successful is whip my dick out."

It could all be so simple, right?

So let's play this game or gayme if you will? You're a LGBTQ black man that wants to make money showing off your dick and possibly have fun with getting paid to have sex with "beautiful people," right? Let's see if you meet the requirements for the "average successful content creator" using social media as their platform to have sex.

As long as you're over five foot four, you need to be weight to height proportion. If you're a big guy, you are going to have to work three times harder if and if you're a top, your stroke game better be A-fuckin'-1. Next, your dick needs to be at least eight and a half inches erect and there is a very strong preference for showers, not growers. The insensitive and irrational audience you're trying to reach wants to already know you have a big dick, not be convinced you can grow one. Don't bring a long pencil dick —you're out. The dick needs to have a nice size girth, with a mushroom head.

Still think it's easy to pull your dick out? Take a few pics and be like "see look, I have a big dick." The problem with that logic is that there are thousands of black men who are physically fit, who can present nice looking eight to twelve inch penises. Anyone can get on the cam after they've taken a shower, stroke their meat, show their hole, and make it enticing. The trick, and this is where a lot of would-be content creators are not successful, is to get the right partners to participate in this game with you. With Atlanta being one of the safest places for black LGBTQ members, there's no accident as to why many of the content creators live within a four hour drive. So it's not entirely impossible to see your favorite content creator in Greensboro, Raleigh, or Charlotte, North Carolina. Nashville, Tennessee, and Birmingham, Alabama are not completely off the map. If we're being honest, it has never been uncommon for people to make the trip from one end of Florida to the other end of Georgia. It helps if you can get a cheap round-trip flight for under $150. Go to Atlanta (or private local with a four hour driving distance), film your content, come home. Make sure you edit that motherfucker, especially if you were scandalous in your encounter. Can't have those corporate logos, family tats or fraternity branding/'nalia showing. The other thing mini content creators are lacking is good promotion. Promotion is not putting your solo flick on Twitter and saying "hey look at me playing with my big black dick. It's about building relationships. It's as simple as saying thank you to the first fifteen to twenty people who give you a compliment. Showing off your interest besides getting naked (gaymers stand up).

***

I finally had him. One of the most prominent men on several adult entertainment sites. He was known for being a man's dream. He was just like the man in the video. Tall, about six foot, smooth dark skin, pretty teeth. His brown skin was a smooth as hard candy, and made me appreciate what India.Aire sang about. His build was perfect for a wide receiver and he moved like a man who commanded attention.

When favorite masculine-presenting sites like DawgPoundUSA, Taggaz and Chocolate Drop were popular, this dude became a well-known, in-demand artist. His dominance as a top that can not only give hard strokes but show a sensual site brought him widespread appeal to mainstream audiences. He equally showed prowess as a bottom that could take strokes as good as he gave them. His most memorable and fan-favorite scenes were the versatile scenes. Fans loved and respected his long-term relationship with a fellow adult video star and appreciated the videos they shared on social media.

"So you're Tony?" He acted like we hadn't talked about this meet up for weeks. I first saw this guy on a few of the popular porn sites. He was a perfectly fit and gifted versatile performer who laid the pipe as well as he took it and his verse scenes were among the best in the industry. On screen, his ass looked impeccable and in person it did not disappoint.

I nodded my head, confirming my identity.

"Show me the money!" He proclaimed as he kicked his shoes off. He didn't have to look too far because the money was on the table where he placed the fitted cap he was wearing. He picked up the $150 that we agreed on, and he left the wallet that was next to it untouched.

"You know you're not getting none of this ass right?"

I hated this condescending tone—I knew the fuckin' rules. He wasn't the first "gay celebrity" I had dealt with. When men who have sex for men solicit services, the price for dick is usually two to three times the price just to suck their dicks. The price for ass was typically ten times the cost for the price of dick or two times their day rate. Over the years, I'd pay for ass and not get it—a lot of these content creators and escorts only want to be topped by the uber wealthy or a man with significant social status.

Or by their peers to promote their fan sites.

I got eight and a half inches and it's a nice width. As I've said before, it works and I'm perfectly capable of topping. I do want to use my dick, but I don't want the pity fucks that come from those who can't get into it with me. I get the psychological issues that come with letting another man penetrate you. The ability to be willing to submit to another man—though truthfully, the bottom has the most power in a gay sex situation, not the top. Very few people are willing to be topped by a man in a chair—even for money.

I've come to accept that.

"I'm good," I replied as I rolled closer to him even though something was triggering my spirit, I still felt at awe being in his presence. I understood what people meant when they said they were mesmerized by a person. This performer was definitely captivating, and had a way of seducing without saying a word. What I didn't like was the cheap cologne he was wearing. I felt like he had just ran into Walmart real quick, sprayed some of the first bottle he could get his hands on and walked out. I wouldn't say he was funky, but this fragrance did not work with his body chemistry.

"How are you getting out of the chair? He asked as he took a seat on my bed, he undressed from the oversized Sean Jean shirt he wore with the matching baggy jeans. Worn some boxer briefs that were them that were made from the same material as biker shorts. That underwear was kind of new at the time and you didn't see too many guys with it.

"I would've liked a little assistance," I was honest as I rolled to the bed. I saw the look of disgust on his face and chose to ignore it because I still wanted this once in a lifetime encounter. "But I can get up. " I use the edge of my bed as a rail and lifted my body out of the chair. Then stretched my arms out to the other end of the bed and pulled my body up.

"Yo, that's nice. Move better than I thought you would," he seemed impressed as he laid across my bed. His penis was flaccid, but still well endowed and not one for disappointment. The dick was a cut thing of beauty and I couldn't wait to fill it in my mouth.

"I can do a lot of things." I spoke confidently as I effortlessly pulled my shirt over my body, then swiftly and quickly lifted my legs up and took off my pants. Again, it would've been nice to get some help, but I could tell that he wasn't the type. Once I got undressed, I immediately put his still soft penis in my mouth, knowing that once I worked my magic, I can get it hard like I can see in the video. It took a few seconds, but I got what I was seeking. As I sucked him, I looked up at him so I could see his face. I was disappointed to see that he had it concealed by his hands. He looked at me, he just saw the look of disappointment in my face.

I stopped sucking him and moved to the side of the bed. I hope he wasn't gonna be one of these limp dick motherfuckers who couldn't perform and still wanted to get paid. I'm not ugly and I wasn't gonna let him treat me as if I was an old rag doll meant to be buried at the bottom of a toy box.

"Can I lay on my back?" I wanted to look at him. Part of the experience I was paying for was to look at the man of my dreams. Also wanted to grab my dick jerk off while he pounded me. He obliged and I'm glad to report that his strokes didn't disappoint. We went from missionary, to me riding him—showing off my gymnastic skills, to him filling up the latex condom as he dawg pounded me on my side.

When he was done, he quickly jumped out of the bed. I turned over in time to notice him rushing to pick up his clothes. I picked up the condom that he left on the bed and saw that my side was clean. I didn't smell any traces of loose bowels or a worn ass smell. When I put the condom down, I did catch him taking the two hundred dollars I'd left in my wallet to go out later this evening out of wallet and into his fitted cap.

"Yo, wassup?!" I yelled out as he grabbed his shoes and ran out of my room butt naked.

I couldn't believe this motherfucker robbed me—nor did I see it coming. I'd felt cheated when I paid money for a twenty minute session and the guy completed in five. But this was the first time I'd been robbed by an escort. I was pissed off but my feelings were hurt more because this guy had everything. Good looks, great body, an equally attractive partner, fame—why steal from me? If he wanted the money, all he had to do was stay another hour or let me top him. Or eat his ass—something. At that time in my life, I would have gladly paid for some more dick rather than go out and be social or pay my bills. My priorities weren't that in order.

I'd gone back and forth over whether or not to disclose the identity of this porn star—notice I said porn star and not content creator. Those of us who watched the black-owned and black leaning studios rise and gain popularity in the early-to-mid 2000's know the difference. I'm choosing not to because once you steal from me, I lose all respect for you. I'm not mentioning the more pleasant interaction I had with his partner or how I tricked off many in his friend group who've admitted he was a fool to steal from me. His name may appear once or twice in the book, but trust it won't be in reference to him. I won't be promoting his business and when people ask about him, I don't send business his way.

Years later, I'm still angered and upset by this, and I deserve better. You could argue that this is the cost of doing business with an escort. There's never the guarantee of getting the service you pay for. It's one thing to be disappointed in the *quality* of the service or to not even get the service. But the blatant in your face the man, that's some fuck shit.

When dealing with escorts and content creators in that way, there is no safety measure to prevent someone from stealing from you. I never know if someone's gonna come in and do what we have agreed or if I'm gonna be assed-out. it's always a risk and gamble and why there are so many warnings not to deal with prostitutes and escorts. In many ways, it is better to just go into an adult bookstore and pay $10-$25 to get in and hope for a good time. That's a gamble too, but you're less likely to be robbed or scammed while in there. More than likely, you'll at least get some head or give some head. If something more happens, then it was a good day. If someone or a group allows you to watch as they do their thing, that's a blessing. If nothing happens as long as you weren't insulted or touched inappropriately, then it's still a good day.

So after this first experience of being robbed by an escort, why would I go back? That is the million dollar question. I know all of them aren't thieves, and despite the drama and incidents I find myself in when dealing with these guys, I still say that I have way more good experiences than bad. Of course, there are some that were disappointing, performance wise, but they didn't steal from me in this position, I've been able to engage many that most of you guys would only just be able to beat your meat to. Some of the guys I've had memorable experiences with that I'll share later in this book and some of the guys, even if we didn't link up sexually, we've become acquaintances. Ironically, some of the guys trust me enough with their mental healthcare and I'm happy for the role that I've been allowed to play in their lives. Others, I've become clients of theirs in their other "professional" endeavors.

These strippers, porn stars, content, creators, and other sexual entertainment workers are people. Very few of them had this and mind as their endgame for when they grow up. Some of the younger ones are just using this as a way to pay for school, much like the young women are allowed to strip to pay for school. I don't think there should be a difference. These guys raise their children, their partners, children, take care of nieces, nephews, and other family members with their bodies. They're active members of various community organizations, mentor young people, and other professionals. They eat, shit and piss the same way we do, some of them have shown you on camera if you're interested.

I endorse these strippers, not as a Barbz (Nicki Minaj fan, guys), but as a proud promoter and participant of the sex work industry. Let these people and other identifying entities get their money, regulate the participants for health and safety reasons and let them pay taxes like any other person.

Just be careful who you let in your home or your body.

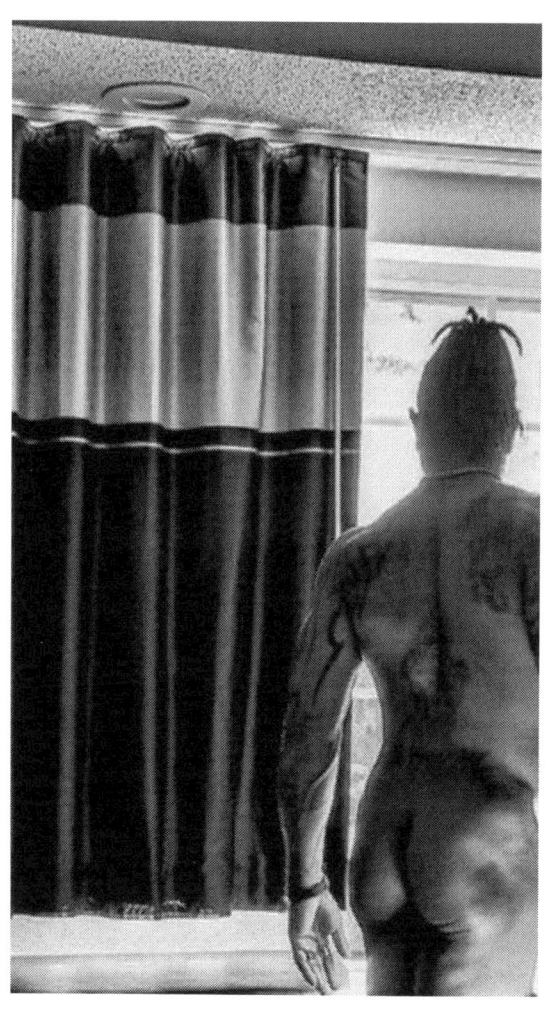

Freakzilla looking out the window.

TOUCH MY BODY

So let's address another elephant in the room, do I, as a physically disabled person deserve to have any physical stimulation that can bring me sexual pleasure?

Hell-fuckin'-yeah.

I deserve to have consensual sexual stimulation whether it's free or I pay for it if I want. I, and every person with special needs should be able to pursue our passions legally and in the manner that we choose. We should not be molested against our will—this happens quite frequently as there are some of us who can't, or won't, speak up for ourselves. That's why I open my big ass mouth because someone needs to tell you about us. Someone got to speak up about the sexual exploitation that happens when we enter relationships, engage in human encounters or pay for services we don't get. Someone has to be brave enough to be the fool. Admit they've been ran over, taken advantage of or abused in some other way.

I'm willing to bet good money I'm not the only one who's been through some of the experiences I've faced. I'm one of the few willing to talk about it publicly.

Or write it in a book.

The audacity and the insult that comes with my sexual liberation and right to interact with others as a viable human being, perplexes me to no end. It's not just the gays that get this shit in their fucking mind, straight people do it, too. This is one thing I think I would experience no matter who I chose to or engage in encounters with me sexually.

Being physically impaired did not and does not control my mental abilities. I can speak English just as well as anyone with a "standard" American education. I received a bachelor's and a master's degree with reasonable accommodations that would be needed because of the need for adaptive technology. Even with writing this book, I dictated portions of it while using speak recognition technology. What Cedric does is type and structure our recorded conversations into text form. He uses his creative writing abilities to pull a book together, recreate stories when needed and formulate a book people would be interested in reading. Then I come behind him and edit the book because I do understand basic and advanced grammar and he's not writing the book himself. I use adaptive technology to read the book to me where needed and like any editor, I pull out my red pen and get to work.

This is my second book with this creator and third overall that I've contributed significantly to that has my name on it. Let's not forget all the papers I've written or helped people write, debates I participate in professionally and socially and other things I can and will do that require a strong mind. I passed several tests to be a licensed therapist in two states, which is my primary source of income at the moment. Not being able to stand and walk did not impact that.

For those of you who have never seen me before, I am technically classified as a paraplegic. I have very limited to no movement of my lower body from the waist down. This does not include the use of my penis or my anus-both perform multiple functions just fine. I was not born a paraplegic, I became one overtime as my cerebral palsy manifested. Cerebral palsy is a neurological disease that affects the body and the brain. Cerebral palsy doesn't take shape in the same way in everyone. For me, it's my lower body that's lost function over time. I used to be able to use walkers, crutches and other walk aids but my legs can't support my weight for long periods of time while standing —definitely not well enough for me to walk. For me, one of the most common outward signs is the fact that at times I may have excessive saliva. I can't help but drool from time to time. As I developed into a young man, my condition played a larger role in the inability to use my legs for longer periods of time. I will admit, some of the reason I can't walk is my fault, because I did not keep up with my walking regimen. It was not for a lack of trying, however.

As a result, I work hard to keep my body in shape. I do exercises that keep my arms strong. I depend on them to help me move, not just carry things. While I can't assist with a traditional lift, I can help lift things up, and hold things up that have a considerable weight. I can move my arms freely, and contrary to operably, if I were to strike at someone with either a punch or a slap, it would come with considerable force behind it. Let me be clear, violence is not my first resort. This is why I use my words so that they may aid me in conflict resolution.

With my hands I can grab, pull, push, grip and move each of my ten fingers independently. Sexually, I can hold a big dick as I'm applying oral pleasure with my mouth. I can twist it, stroke it and do anything any other man or woman can do. I can grab my own dick with either hand and bring myself to completion. I can finger myself and bring about stimulation from my prostate. My upper body dexterity has been my biggest strength when it comes to having sex. Just as easily as I can do a push up on the floor or a pull up if the bar is low enough for me to reach from my chair; I can hold, pin down, touch and caress. My fingers tickle, grip a dick, twist and turn in a nigga's ass. My physical disability doesn't affect my hands and the way I can make you feel. Even with lower body dexterity, I can still do some things. I can be propped up on a wall and you could bounce on my dick that way. I can be ridden in my wheelchair.

The tricky part is getting on my knees. I can't elevate my upper body and be fully supported or comfortable. I can do the basics like move my legs, wiggle my toes—I can feel my feet. I can be penetrated doggy style, because I have great upper body dexterity, my arms are able to support the position. If you were to wrap my legs around you while thrusting into me in the missionary position, I would need help keeping my legs around your waist. However, if you fold me back or twist me like a pretzel, my legs will go wherever you want them to go. I can be penetrated from the side as long as you hold up one of my legs for better access. Contrary to popular belief, I can be fucked "standing" up. That would require me leaning on a sturdy base or being able to grip a bar very tightly. You have to be right on me and to a point be able to support my weight. I can bounce on a dick in any position provided there is a sturdy base that either I can lift up and down with my arms or if you are moving my waist up and down as if I were a life-sized masturbator.

The problem with having sex with me, is that people don't wanna *touch my body*. I need what Mariah sings about in the chorus of her song. I don't understand why people won't touch me because I'm not fragile. You have to touch the person you are being intimate with, no matter how you are stimulating them. Most of my escorts prefer that they just lay on their back or I put a comforter or pillow over my face while they are drilling me, pretending that I'm someone else. Excuse me, you rude motherfuckers, but this is *my* experience. I'm paying for this! I need my nipples to be twisted, pinched, and flicked. It would be nice if my body was rubbed. Massages would be great while I'm getting back strokes. I like my dick played with no matter how I'm being penetrated. Get me off. That's what I'm paying for. If you can do it for others, then dammit, do it for me.

Part of the reason you were chosen to stimulate me, it's not just because I crave intimacy. You were chosen so that I could have a full encounter and experience *with you*. So my advice to all the people who think they want to get into escorting and want to make this as a side career to their social media, profiles, dancing, and other things that support their content creation is treat the consumer right. Whether you like it or not I, the John, am the customer. We're not all gonna look like rappers or movie stars or undercover, discreet athletes. Your John's come in all shapes and sizes. And no matter how we earn our money, when you get it, it will all spend the same.

I'll let you in on a little secret, some of your Johns talk, just as much as y'all talk to other escorts. So that appointment that got canceled at the last minute, could be a result of a John hearing about a terrible experience with you. The nasty attitudes that you display on social media, the fighting you do amongst yourself, the inability to get hard both on and off camera, all of this affects your money. Scamming and robbing your clients isn't the best choice of action and karma will catch that ass, eventually.

Consider this, the average adult performer has a career that spans two to three years. It can last longer if they make content that either "goes viral," or, they're able to produce a massive amount of content and have complete ownership and control of said content. A pretty face, a nice body, a big dick, and a fat ass will not keep you in business long-term. The smart ones who do research on Twitter or Instagram before they engage in this activity find most adult performers have other interests besides sex. In fact, I respect that quite a few of them have successful careers outside of porn, and oddly enough, the most successful ones use adult entertainment as a side gig and something fun to do. That's probably why they make the most money, they don't need it. It's been my experience that these guys often are the best when it comes to escorting. These types of escorts do this because they get pleasure out of seeing whoever they're penetrating get pleasure. That's what turns them on.

I could reference countless other people who've had what appears to be great chemistry on camera, but conflicts off camera. There's a reason why some of your "favorite performers" don't work together. What may not be publicly known is that some of them are blood relatives so they're not gonna practice incest for your pleasure. That's just a small minority. What is known, and what the camera catches is the lack of chemistry between two performers. Watch a video and you know ol'boy's dick is not hard. The two performers are going through the motions. The scenes are mediocre.

The same performance these guys give on screen gets worse when they come to us. They want $100 to $200 to bring half-hard dicks or pieces they require drugs for (which I'm gonna address in another section of the book). They come to us rank from the funk that went beyond the workout, dancing or sexing a precious John. It's downright atrocious. Yet some of us put it aside because we want to be touched or pleasured.

There are John's that settle for mediocrity just so they can feel intimacy with another individual.

That's me, I'm that individual.

Of course, I could demand more because even though I have physical needs, I deserve more. It's not low self-esteem that keeps me in this rut where I put up with abuse, defamation of character or just random bullshit most of you wouldn't put up with from a regular motherfucker. I think my situation is deeper than that. I've grown accustomed to the mistreatment and I've tricked my spirit into believing there is nothing else.

My spirit believes I don't deserve better…sometimes.

When I catch myself going too far I do what I need to do to pull myself back up. Even I'm not immune to the tricks of the mind.

That's when I call on the next escort, and hope he can do it better than the last one.

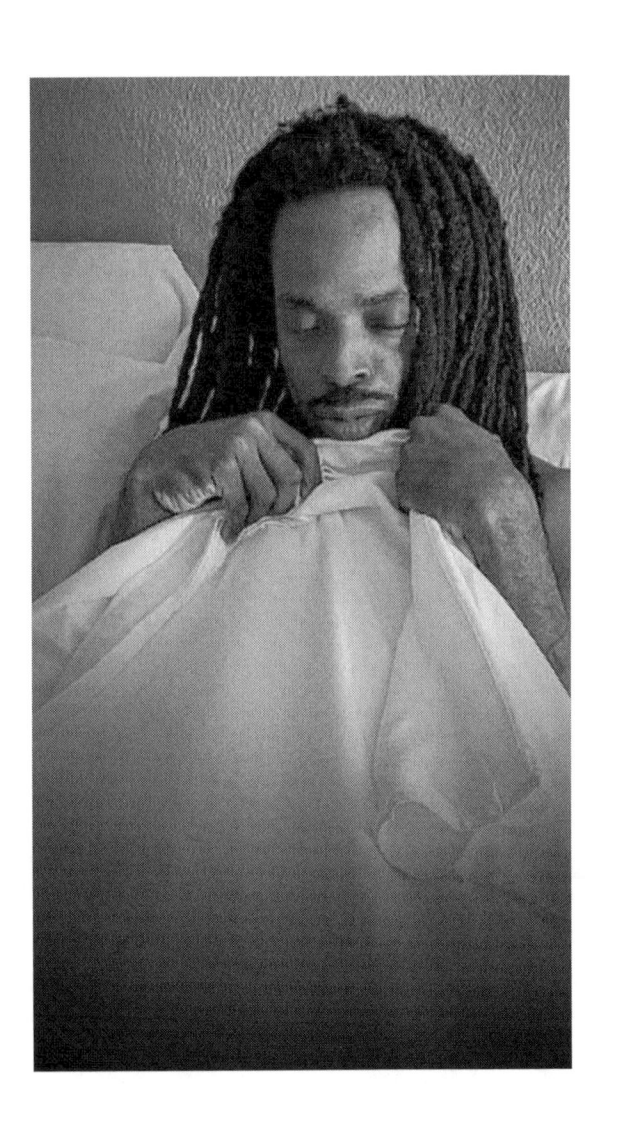

MAGIC STICK

Forrest Gump's quote about life and chocolates can also apply to dicks. Every man is packing one–but they aren't all the same. I can't look at a man and say "ooh, he's gonna have a big dick" or just because he's hung like a banana doesn't guarantee that I'm gonna get a good experience.

The first time I saw a penis after puberty was in the locker room in high school. I didn't gawk with my eyes bulging like an animated cartoon character, I acknowledged to myself "oh, his dick looks nice," and went about my business getting dressed. When I was young and had no business sneaking and watching my brother's porn collection and magazines–that's when I lusted after the sheer beauty of all those chocolate-colored dicks inside of those pretty pink pussies. When the ladies got'em wet or the guys rubbed their spit, lube or other secretions to make them shine, that's when I got on cloud nine.

I don't feel like I was overexposed to dick, but seeing and feeling as many as I have had, has made me come to appreciate dick for what it is. We all know that its primary anatomical call function is to release urine and human waste from the body. Its secondary function is to contribute to the reproduction of life. As men, we need both of those things to fully function, and for many of us our penises, become a part of our masculine identity. Like every boy my age, I'm guilty of trying to hijack Cinemax or Showtime to see if I could catch a glimpse of some peen. I'd be disappointed because all I saw were white women, pretending to be bouncing on flaccid penises. Their kitties flopping around like uncoordinated yo-yos. The gazing, pretending to be in lust while trying to hide a snicker. The dancing, grinding—sometimes through static did nothing but get me in unnecessary trouble if the sound was louder than I thought it was when I flipped to the channel.

HBO—them motherfuckers knew what the fuck they were doing. *Oz* kept me up and satisfied. I want to give a shout out to all the actors who showed their actual flaccid dicks without using a body double. Watching *Oz* played a role in how I came to accept my body—don't get it twisted. I watched *Oz* for its gritty and graphic storyline as much as I did to see the random man or men naked. No one can have a show past one season if all you got to offer is ass and dick. When I went to the movies or was able to rent them from Blockbuster, I loved seeing Allen Payne, Taye Diggs, Mario Van Peoples, Omar Epps getting them draws because they always kept mine wet. *Real Sex, Taxicab Confessions, The Wire and Arliss* kept me busy.

I'm glad that HBO had a hold on me because seeing the variety of dicks I saw on that channel helped me understand that we're not all built the same and that we don't all work the same. Just as much as I enjoyed seeing the meat swinging without having to watch a porn (another plus for the network), I liked hearing some of the men talk about infertility, erectile dysfunction, size insecurity. All of those things made the men who were on those shows relatable to me. Being in a wheelchair, people assume that bottoming is my only role and that my dick doesn't work.

For one, my dick does a better job getting hard than a twenty year old who's on Tina—and it's bigger, too. It's nice and cut—I got a good mushroom head. It's five inches flaccid, eight when erect and it's as thick as an air freshener can. Curves slightly to the left—it's not the biggest but definitely one of the prettiest.

The old Black Men (Blackmen.com/Blackmen4now.com) and BGCLive websites made me appreciate the cartoons and the models who showed off their dicks in various stages of erection. I didn't always get an erection when I saw a juicy plump dick I wanted to suck. A lot of times, I could appreciate being able to see the work of art. On days I was bold, I'd contact and continue conversation with the model or artist if there was an invitation to do so.

I can tell you what any man or woman who'd ever had a dick inside of them will tell you—they don't all feel the same. Yes, they're flesh and blood and fulfill a certain need. The owner, in many cases, determines what kind of dick he's going to have or what kind of dick he's going to give you. Athleticism is attractive oftentimes because it's assumed they are going to have the firmest and stiffest pieces of meat out there. Many times they do—but if they can't dance, they can't stroke. Even that's not a guarantee. I've had fat boys pull out nine inches like it's nothing—bet they'd have twelve or close to it if their FUPA's didn't get in the way. I've had skinny boys make baby carrots look monstrous. Like I said earlier, you never know with these things.

What I wish most men knew was how to take care of their dicks. We have guys who still think taking a bath twice or three times a week is good or who don't know how to take a rag (if they use one) and wash the crack of their ass. Bro, washing your ass and your dick is not going to make you gay—having good hygiene will determine if I suck your dick and how long. I'm not saying shave or trim your pubes, but if I can smell your body odor when you pull your pants down, imagine what your dick smells like. Come on bros, you know you can smell the rankness of unwashed dead skin cells on your ball sacks.

I DON'T WANT TO SUCK ON THAT!!!

I wouldn't say put baby powder or cologne (which makes it worse in some cases) down there but if you know we are going to hook up—especially if I'm calling and paying you for your service, don't bring me no rank dick. No, "I just worked an eight hour shift and I haven't had time to shower yet," dick—if you do, expect to jump in the tub before you do anything with me. Take care of your dick —seeing a urologist is not a bad thing if you know you are having problems. Don't wait until the last minute before it's too late.

I do want to say that black men, we are more than our dicks. For centuries, we've been thought of as meat factories. In the Americas, we were used to populate and produce new workers cheaply. Then when we got a little bit of freedom, evil white people who hung us from trees would cut the penises off, put them in boxes and pass our manhood down their generations as proof of the work they done. White women would lie on our dicks, accuse them of rape and cause mass murders that have yet to be atoned for. Now, everyone wants to see them in person. On a plate or the print in the gray sweatpants.

But here's my question—what happens when you got to meet the man beyond the dick? Don't get me wrong, a dick feels good when a man knows how to use it, but what about the man the dick is attached to? I typically don't mess with men who I know are married—and if I do and I'm aware in advance, I get the spouse's consent. You'd be surprised at not only how many of them say yes, but actively support their men making money with their dicks. I don't want men that come with too many baby mamas, too much debt, no job or have no ambition. Even for a fuck buddy, that's not going to do it for me. No one's dick is good enough for me to switch gears mid-shift. If we agree to $100 then we agree to $100. I try to avoid problematic dick but sometimes, I can't avoid it. I don't find out the dick is abusive until after it's been inside of me. After the fist connected to the dick's owner landed in my face. After I've been kicked out of a moving vehicle (that's happened more than once) or after the dick has burned me.

In the grand scheme of things, the seven to twelve inches I deal with all get me to a point—not just something that moves and tantalizes one of my holes but brings me a level of intimacy. The cuddling after we've both climaxed is often more fun than the sex itself. How many songwriters have said "I'm looking for somebody I can talk to."

Shit, me too.

Dick is good, real good. But in order to have the "Magic Stick" that 50 and Kim rap about, it's gotta have more than length, girth, good features (a hood is optional). It's gotta have all its correct functions. Most importantly, its owner has got to be the total package. Whether I'm paying for companionship or in a relationship, the dick has to do more than get hard to satisfy me.

SEX & CANDY

The first time someone told me that poppers were VHS video head cleaners, I almost gagged. I knew then in all my life I had seen and heard it all. We've reached a point where anything can be turned into a drug to get off.

I don't know if poppers were around all my life but lately, it would appear that many men carry them around like they were a fresh stick of gum. Gotta smell that alcohol-like aroma that gets the boys horny. I know bottoms that say it makes it easier to take dick and tops who think it keeps the dick harder.

I always thought the phrase sex and candy was weird and when I looked up what John Wozinak meant when he wrote the song, I laughed. Sex and candy would be the perfect explanation to the modern day male on male sexual experience.

When dudes aren't inhaling poppers, they're into the real drugs. Marijuana doesn't bother me much but it's the guys that do Tina that keep the drama going. Tina is slang for crystal methyl. They put it in a glass pipe, light the bulb and inhale the smoke. When consumed it leaves a burnt wire smell and is frequently used at sex parties for male to male activity.

If I believed the social media hookup sites, everyone was on T. I would see parTy (yes, it's spelled right) in several profiles. Puts a whole new spin on Jagged Edge's "Where the Party At".

Not in my room. I go through enough taking regular drugs for my Cerebral Palsy, HIV and Herpes. I don't need to add illicit drugs that could cause me to lose what body functions I have to the list.

In a foolish move, I gave a popular adult performer, who I will not name, a chance when he was on T. The way he said it was "a *different* kind of high" was an understatement. Would've thought I was listening to Lil Kim. Like most guys who saw his videos where he was giving and getting dick, I wanted to see if he could live up to the hype. He promised that if I sent his reduced fee and covered his drugs, I'd experience the best I ever had.

Okay Drake, making promises. I wanted the experience and admittedly, I'd never been with a guy on T before. Before I go any further, I must state that consent from both parties was obtained while we both were sober. I was physically with this person when we arranged this encounter and from what I know, he was not drunk, had not smoked and I had no reason to believe he was by any means incapacitated.

I went with it and within two hours, he had what he needed and we were going to proceed. It didn't take me long to prep on my end because while I didn't anticipate an encounter, I wanted to stay ready because I had someone else I wouldn't have to pay lined up the next day.

We got into the bed and he was still smoking on the pipe. I touched his flaccid member and it felt like I had homemade slime in my hand. It was worse than a limp noodle because that penis had no texture at all. I felt like if I tugged at the tip of his dick hard enough, the whole thing would have detached from his body. I tried stroking him, hoping that if I gave him some good head, he could grow in my mouth.

Nothing happened.

"Turn over," he commanded.

I did so willingly hoping that him grinding on me better than Pretty Ricky would do the trick. Damn he was pretty, but Ricky disappointed as he couldn't get it up. He tried to stuff it in on soft and do a few pumps but I lowered myself on the bed and turned around.

"You're not getting hard," I wanted to cry because once again, I played myself for a damn fool.

"Why don't you suck on it again?" He pleaded. I wanted my money back. What it look like not being able to swallow Jell-O? That's exactly what putting his dick in my mouth would do. Piss me the fuck off.

We tried watching a scene of Aye Papi banging out some pretty nigga from DawgPoundUSA but he couldn't pound me with a noodle dick. I was so mad–I wanted to kick his ass. I wanted my money back but he smoked some of it. "I'm sorry." He murmured as he got up and put his pants back on.

"I want my money back!" I demanded as I tried to be cordial as he rushed to finish getting dressed. He grabbed his drugs and his backpack and made a dash for the door. I wanted to yell, scream. I can't believe this bitch ass dude tricked me out of my money.

"I want my money back!" I yelled as I rushed to wrap the sheet around my waist. I hustled to my chair and strapped my legs into the braces of my wheelchair. This fucker was out the door but I was determined to catch him. I snapped the seat belt around my waist and rolled to the spot on the floor where my shirt was. I forgot in my rush to catch this guy that I couldn't reach down and grab my shirt without a grabber stick or something to lift the shirt up. I decided that it would be in my best interest to leave the shirt and roll after him so I could get some help. I'd already been robbed one time and I didn't want this to become a repeat event.

By time I got to the door, I had no clue as to where he went. There was no trace of the Tina he smoked to give me a clue which way he went. Be my damn luck, he had a getaway driver waiting in the cut, ready to help him escape.

I tried not to get mad at myself but I could've sworn I had learned this lesson already. Either way, I guess I should be happy he didn't physically hurt me. My feelings, my pride and my money were gone, but at least I'm still here. Should be thankful.

I will say, I learned this lesson and I made sure that I never dealt with a guy who does drugs again. Sex and candy–both tasted bitter to me.

SEX ROOM

For some, one option to bypass all the fuckery that comes with the escorts and prostitution is to go to a venue that has an adult theater, glory holes and other amenities.

The venues are sometimes called bookstores, sex stores, hot spots, day motels, etc. One thing in common is that they have theaters in various rooms. Some show straight videos, others show gay, lesbian and transgender porn. Every now and then the specialty video comes on.

The venues are not exclusive to gay or bisexual men—though it's known and understood that it is the gay and bisexual dollar that keeps the venues open. Single men who want to have "adult happy fun time" as Nico Aesthetics would call it, pay the premium to go to the theaters, which are safe "cruising" spots. "Cruising" in the gay sex world is when a man walks around a public place that are "underground hangout spots" to meet other men in which arrangements can be made to have consensual sex at another location (or a secret location at that spot). In the venues, "cruising" is done in order to get another guy or two to meet and have a sexual encounter in a booth or in a private room in the theater. The private rooms typically cost a premium in addition to entry into the spot and the renter is given a pass or key for a certain amount of hours.

Fair warning, not all places allow or condone sexual acts to be performed on the premises—in many localities, states and countries, the acts are against the law.

On the onset, many aren't handicapped accessible but have found unique ways to make those of us in chairs feel part of the community. Some will pull out makeshift ramps and others will let us in back door entrances if permitted. A lot of the places I've been to will go out of their way to welcome a handicapped person and make them feel wanted in their space.

Entry into these places usually are granted to those eighteen and up and many of these places card everyone prior to admission—so be prepared to show a valid state issued license or ID or a federal passport. Once admittance has been granted, it's good to be aware that the venues have a lot of written and unwritten rules. The obvious written ones are:

1. One person per booth.
2. No urinating or defecating in the booth.
3. Clean up after yourself.
4. Do not break anything—if you do, be prepared to replace it.
5. Be respectful of other patrons.

6. Only engage in conversation or physical touch with consent.

Some places have their own rules about:
1. How long admission to the theater lasts.
2. If re-entry is allowed and how to acquire access to that.
3. What can or cannot happen in their parking lot.
4. What's considered "their" property.

It's best to follow these rules because breaking them can get you banned from their stores and even rival bookstores. Doesn't seem fair but why would Venue B want to deal with you if you were a problem at Venue A and/or Venue C? It would suck to travel and know that you can't enter a venue in Atlanta cause of some foolishness they found out you did in Dallas or St. Louis.

Word travels.

As far as unwritten rules go, the biggest is that "no" means "no." No. A complete sentence. Regardless of what happens, "no" needs to be understood as the ultimate safe word. All action stops. Anything that happens after "no" can be considered sexual assault. This rule applies to men and women and from what I've witnessed, the management of these places typically are consistent when enforcing this rule.

Another unwritten rule is that if there is a couples' room, the women run the shop. Not all venues have couples' rooms–during events, typically the "straight rooms" are designated couples' rooms for these events. On the popular couples' nights, the woman, who is usually accompanied by a man, can kick single men out of the room in certain venues and designated nights. Along with this rule is that couples can decide that certain spaces or rooms are couples' only when they are present. Usually, in order for this to work, there has to be at least two couples present. I've seen situations where four couples entered their portion of the room, selected four single men to participate and kicked everyone else out. On nights like this, straight men either know not to come or they walk around the hallways, hoping not to be approached by a gay man wanting to cruise. Or they talk in the smoking areas in hopes that a couple stopping by chooses them to engage in some shenanigans. Most of the time, the women like to watch and be watched—a few like to participate—and a few get turned on by watching their men get handled. The only places they cannot outright take over are the designated gay spaces. If two men are fucking in the gay theater, they can't make them stop because they want the couch or the couples' room is full.

While it's known that gay sexual acts do happen in the "straight rooms", anyone can ask for homosexual sex, whether it's between two men or two women, to stop in the "straight room." One of the few unwritten rules that benefit men because no one should be forcibly subjected to sexual acts they do not wish (or do not have consent) to participate in. Yes, lesbian and bisexual women do have to stop acts in a "straight room" if they aren't willing to let a single man participate.

Every venue has their own written and unwritten rules —those that patronize the place will fill you in if they catch you doing something amiss.

One of the most important things is to be respectful. These places are the only safe haven a few of us have to be sexually free. Be safe, have fun and get it in.

To be honest, I only go to adult bookstores sparingly. It's not that I dislike the places. Actually, I would promote and recommend everyone try them. For the purposes of this book, I will not list specific places, only to tell you to do your research and ask around. People on the popular dating apps will tell you where to go.

The pros about the venues are that when I step into one, I can be whoever I wanna be. I come prepared for what I want to do, and there is an expectation that I have body autonomy. If I want to top, all I gotta do is whip my dick out, show that it can stay hard, and somebody will bounce on it. Being in this chair almost makes me a circus attraction. No, don't think that I think that I'm a weirdo, but I'm the new freak in town. A lot of people admire the fact I have the balls to roll my ass up in the damn store to begin with. So, like I said, whip my dick, I get it hard, and eventually somebody's gonna suck on it. Somebody's gonna ride it. I'm gonna be played with and it's those moments where I feel like I'm part of the community.

I've had a freaky bottom or two try to spin my chair around as they rode me like a mechanical bull. A fuckin' thrill. The guy who tried to make my chair do hydraulics almost broke my chair but props for trying to make the most out of my chair. Needless to say, I've had memorable topping experiences there, that I appreciate if for no other reason, allowing me to explore my versatile side. And I get fucked there, too. I've had a guy take me out of the chair, put me on the bench, strip butt naked, get in my chair, and have me ride him. This fine ass thugged-out, Mexican had me bouncing on his pinga like I was in a Rhyheim Shabazz video.

Sometimes, I go to the stores to have another sexually active person to talk to. I get to openly and plainly talk about what I like and don't like sexually and people want to hear more of my story. I wouldn't say that I'm popular but a venue is one place where I feel like I belong. I don't have to deal with the pretty boy privilege, and Insta/social media faggot drama. I get to be who I am authentically.

And the guys are with it or they're not. At least in these spaces, if a guy is not interested in me, they're respectful about it.

I think Annie Lennox said it best, "everybody's looking for something." It doesn't have to be me, but I do like that I'm in a rather safe environment to try something new. To a degree when I'm in a bookstore I'm in a safe space where I shouldn't have to worry about being assaulted. Most of these places don't have security, but because most of the patrons respect what these venues provide, many people abide by the rules.

I'm not oblivious to the disadvantages. I know I'm not everybody's cup of tea, so I'm often not chosen for the everyday sexual experience, and I'm okay with that. That doesn't mean that I'm left unattended because somebody wants to try me out. I can't stand up long enough to put my dick through the glory hole so I can't get my dick sucked that way. I've had someone try to fuck me that way and it didn't work. That means that sometimes when people want to have encounters with me they either have to leave the door open, or we have to do it out in the open. I'm not really the kind of person who wants public sex—I do it sometimes because in the moment, I'm comfortable.

One of the reasons that I prefer to pay well-known performers hundreds of dollars versus the typical $10-$20 entry fee. Many of these places charge around the country is because I know what I'm getting. When I link up with a random, I never know what to expect. As I've said before, I don't go to these places often enough to be a regular or to know who is a regular. Sometimes, I will be the second or third person I've seen a top with because I've seen them work other people. Then it's having to tell people in an open space "I'm HIV positive and I have herpes." Not to mention that I don't prefer condoms, but I will wear one when I'm in these spaces. While most people appreciate my honesty, just as many don't give a fuck, and they're probably in the same situation.

In researching for this book, Cedric and others, who asked to remain anonymous, shared some of their experiences with me. It's interesting to see how these places work based on race, age, sexual preference, and other distinguishing factors. There are days when big boys are the flavor of the night and others when it's "white boys only." There is a general preference for "fit boys" and the gym rats are chased around and even offered money to participate. In general, it's the average, everyday man that goes in there. With his average five to seven inch dick–looking for something, be it mouth, ass or pussy to stick. While some may make arrangements to hook up in advance, many take the gamble. Admission is like playing an expensive lottery ticket–at minimum, getting (or giving) some head is almost the equivalent to getting your money's worth. A hand job is like losing some money but not leaving empty handed. Fucking is the jackpot. Better than coffee in the morning or whatever it was Miguel said.

ME, MYSELF AND I

Confession…I don't like sex toys.

No, don't be mad. It's just that I feel like the toys are so impersonal. I've always been accustomed to the touch and feel of a real man. Even if I had to pay for it, that was better than nothing.

Let me clarify when I say that it's not that I don't use toys. When I have a choice, they're not my "go to" for sexual satisfaction. Whether I'm using a masturbator on my dick, or a dildo in my ass, a lot of the toys are a lot of work for me to have to use them either to prep or for "pleasure. " For one, most of the toys require that I'm out of my chair on the bed or laying down on the floor. Then I got to use my hand to move the toy in and out of my cavity. Why am I preparing myself when I'm not getting the real thing?

Structurally, toys aren't built to be used in a chair, and discriminatory, toys are designed for fully functioning people. In my opinion, the ideal sex toy would be one that requires less hassle to use while I'm in a chair. I don't wanna have to shift and move my body in such a way in order for the toy to work. I shouldn't have to make any adjustments or secure my chair in a particular way. I know it seems like I'm asking for a lot, but this is one way that people with needs are excluded from the sex conversation. And by no means am I faulting the toy manufacturers, because they are thinking about the majority of the people who are not in chairs, not using walkers, and like to do the freaky shit that I can't do in my chair. I can imagine that if a toy were designed for me to use safely, it would be very, very expensive. I can also imagine it would be very heavy, because for a paraplegic or even someone who is wheelchair bound for the majority of their time, the toy has to be sturdy for us to maneuver on it or around it.

However, let me just say that it's not that you shouldn't try to, nor am I taking a dig at those of you who find toys enjoyable. I'm saying that I don't like them, for me. I'm open to trying many different toys as they come out. I'm even open to being on a panel where if people with physical needs were thought of, we could test out toys and give our input on how the toys would be better for us. Maybe I'm looking in the wrong place or have put as much thought into this, but when I searched different toys, there are very few toys that I would say are ADA Friendly for someone with my specific physical disabilities.

I will say that cock rings aren't too bad. They take some getting used to and I see why guys wear them, whether they're topping and jacking off, or receiving the pounding. The right cock ring has a nice grip around your balls and hits the taint area just right. It's a nice feeling, almost like a glove. I like wearing the vibrating ones where you can tuck the vibrator under your scrotum, and it massages your prostate. It has an additional sensation when you're being penetrated from the back and ironically, it tends to loosen you up when you take bigger dicks. For me when you wear the vibrator on top of your shaft, it tickles. It is a good pulsating, filling that encourages you to thrust as you're delivering strokes or jacking your meat.

The body mannequins and body masturbators are either too light or too heavy to use. The blowup dolls are cute to look at and they are entertaining. Sometimes I get a good laugh, especially when I see people use them on television. Realistically, the dildos attached to them aren't designed for anal penetration. There's too much work involved when I would have to ride it, or commit to a reverse cowgirl position With the blowup dolls, I'd have to worry about them deflating which can inadvertently cause the makeshift dildo to cause harm to my anal cavity. With the heavier, weighted dolls I'm missing the human touch. A doll can't smack my ass, smack my face, twist my dick, or talk shit to me while I'm riding. And a doll can't do it doggy style. I could get one of those machines that poked me, but if the machine malfunctions, it would cost a lot to fix. Not to mention the heaviness of being able to pick the machine up and the assistance I may need in setting it up. I will admit that dolls can serve a purpose of giving the simulation of laying next to someone.

Dildos are my biggest problem. Not all of them are created equal and not all of them provide the pleasure I want to have when participating in anal sex. However, I want to talk about oral sex first. They're okay to practice sucking a dick on. It's cute to be able to get the multi-striped ones that measure "how far you can go." In my opinion, the suckers that are shaped like penises, serve a better purpose for that. They typically leave a better taste in my mouth and don't have the strange aftertaste that you can get from the different types of plastics and silicone that are used. Plus the right flavored dildo can be more encouraging to pursue greater less, if you catch my drift.

Then with dildos, it's sometimes the size, shape, and color. Since I like real dicks, I naturally prefer a dildo that is shaped like a real penis. I wish there were improvements and creating shafts so that we can have uncut dildos in addition to cut dildos. Perhaps an uncut dildo could teach the boys that don't know how to clean their penises correctly how to do so. Get under the hood and clean boys. Roll it over, wipe and clean, roll it back, wipe and clean. For those of us who like the feel of uncut dick in our asses, the extra skin that gives you that extra tickle when it's being thrust inside of you for a more memorable and realistic sensation. I don't like the tubed or weird shaped vibrators that women are able to use. I think because of how a vagina is designed those dildos are not designed for anal pleasure, and you even have to be careful with using them for oral pleasure as they can cause unintended injuries.

I do like dildos that are realistic in size. Six to nine inches could typically satisfy me for every day or frequent usage. I like that real men and famous adult content creators are able to get cast moldings of their penises and are able to market and sell them. I can see how using the dildo, while watching the video of the performer creates more of the illusion of actually having sex with that performer. Amount those in my demographic, PhatRabbitKiller's (PRK) toy is a go to. It's as close as most people are gonna get to having him. Anton Harden, Rob Piper, Jax Slayher, Alex Jones, Isaiah Maxwell, Brickzilla, Damion Dayski, Mr. Marcus, Dredd, Prince Yashua, Sean Michaels are all the black performers that have toys made from their dicks (thank you IceKreammFreek for the X/Twitter post).

Some people like to watch the videos of the performer that they have a dildo of. The imagination is strong and it's easy to pretend like you're the bottom getting fucked instead of the guy on the video. I've never gotten to do this, but I've seen videos where people have posted themselves using the dildos while listening to the performer's video in the background.

When I first was pursuing escorts for sexual services, I looked into ballroom and the chat lines because that's what I had available to me. Through them, I gained access to well-known porn stars and those who had memorable scenes in videos. Pornography was good for providing sounds to stimulate me while I masturbated or a good visual for an image I could store in my mind. I eventually started using porn to seek out performers to make my fantasies come true.

I look at the guys in the videos and before fan sites became popular, I'd stream the videos on famous adult content sites or I'd get DVDs from a local salesman. I'd watch a few and when I get the performer's information, I'd be able to reference what they'd done in a particular video for what I wanted in my session. Porn made it easier to articulate what I wanted because I already had the evidence that they could do the desired task. With social media, direct contact made the performers more accessible. Certain payment platforms made it easier to tip them to get their attention.

Porn provided a safe way to view the guys I wanted to see in sexual situations and wanted to have sex with. I watched it in the comfort of my own home and no one knew my preference unless they saw my video stash or had access to my computer. Let's not get it twisted, porn doesn't automatically get my dick hard or my pants wet. With adult content being readily accessible through a variety of platforms, I can't afford to get hard or have sex on the brain every time some good looking dick comes across the screen. I may have watched so much of it, I've learned to restrain and control my desires. I have to be in a certain mood and a particular setting to be aroused by porn.

With access to so many stars, I've almost become desensitized to the erotic effects of a naked black man on the screen. It's like the opposite effect of watching too much porn. Instead of not being able to handle or deal with the human touch, watching porn is like watching another television show. I log in, get a good laugh, watch to see if the models do anything I haven't seen them do before, then I log off. Contrary to popular belief, I don't always use porn as a modern day catalog to find men. What happens is if I see a few of your scenes and I'm tuned in enough to want to touch myself, I'd rather just spend the money to have them. I reach out, find out their price, and after a few weeks of communication, either a link up happens, or it doesn't. A lot of times I lose interest if the model can't hold simple conversation and answer basic question. At this stage in the game, you should know if you're interested in even doing sex work with paying clients. I do get told that some models only perform with other models, and I accept that answer because everyone has a right to choose. Some have told me they don't find me attractive, and they'd rather not scam me then force themselves to pull off the act. I'd rather be told that with the intention of being no harm, no foul, then for someone to try to bait me along to see what kind of money they can get out of me, and have no intention to do right with me.

Interacting with these models, I'm realize that content creators and porn stars are human. I've never seen them as being anything less than, but I think in the gay culture, porn stars are elevated to a celebrity status in a way that they aren't in straight culture. We also erroneously assume that if a content creator or gay porn star has done "a lot of videos," that also means "they have a lot of money." There are a lot of broke, porn stars and content creators. Some use sex work in its various forms as a side hustle while maintaining regular 9 to 5 jobs. Some are battling addictions, and/or don't know how to manage their money which contributes to the troubles they find themselves in.

People waiting for new content from their favorite creators are worse than people who live their lives around when the next pair of Jordans come out. Lotta times these content creators film content that they can use for a later date. The smart ones schedule their releases so they can insure their multiple videos are cut and edited correctly to produce the best content possible. My favorite content creators have regular regular partners they film with. I like that I can always depend on a video with content creator A and content creator B at least 2 to 3 times a year. The chemistry is always there, and I know that every time content creator A and content creator B film together. they're always going to give me a good scene. In today's world, you can come up with your own combination that this sentence would apply for.

My biggest challenge has not been coming up with the content creator's rate, booking a flight or getting them to stay with me an extended period of time. It has been being able to book two of them at the same time for a threesome. Because I use so many of them I'm somewhat privy to who doesn't like who, personal or professional problems between different creators, and in some cases, who's related. I'm not going to expose that here, but I would say the main reason I've been unable to fulfill this dream of mine has fallen into one of these three categories.

I can always update this book if I fulfill this fantasy.

I've considered being a content creator, myself. A part of me thinks that I would be a good representation with those of us who do have physical disabilities that we are dealing with. I believe in porn that there's a market for everyone. I wouldn't go as far as to say that anyone can be a star, but I can say that for every skin tone, there's a fetish for it. People are interested in people of different shapes, sizes, age groups, occupations, and even twisted fantasies, some of which are legal. But the sheer diversity of kinks and pleasures does leave adult content, creation, wide open. Of course, I do have a particular type that I want to perform with, but I'm also mature enough to understand that I don't fit into everyone's cross market. I'd only want to film with those whom I feel safe with and can help me get the job done. I'd also have to do quite a bit of work building my audience, and at this moment in my life, that's not something I'm truly interested in doing. I don't think you should enter porn, content creation, or any other endeavor if you're not genuinely motivated to see it through. or do it right.

Maybe one day I will. Hell, many of you have already seen me naked. With as much money as I have paid and spent in porn and escorting, I should consider being on the other side.

We'll see.

PILLS N POTIONS
(CEDRIC QUINCY PREP INTERLUDE)

When I first heard about a pill that would help men who were HIV negative be able to stay that way, I was excited and nervous. Excited because my next thought was *we are one step closer to a cure.* One step to being able to remove the stigma that HIV has placed on the black community. Nervous because I wondered how much the medication would cost. Without the generosity of donors and special programs from the government and pharmaceutical companies, many people would not be able to afford to pay the *true* cost of medications. I remember when the cocktail of HIV medications were over five thousand a month, which was not obtainable to the average person who was positive.

To be fair, HIV treatment and medications were not the only ones that were expensive. I've had partners who took very expensive treatments for heart disease, neuropathy, seizures and other illnesses I won't disclose here. I dreaded paying up to five hundred dollars out of pocket each month for their pills and potions. As I now work to manage my own issues with blood pressure and weight loss, I'm grateful that my medications aren't as costly–but I couldn't imagine having to pay for my treatments without medical insurance. Which brings about a different stress–staying at a job because you need the insurance to make the medication affordable.

Aside from the costs, the mental strain that came with testing for HIV. I dreaded the calls/texts/messages from a partner or medical facility notifying me that I had been exposed to the virus and needed to get tested immediately. Some of the partners who helped me get in this position would duck and dodge me. At the time, I often worked jobs where I had no health insurance and as a small business owner that was still finding my footing, I couldn't afford the expensive premiums because I wasn't part of a group plan. While I lived in one metropolitan city in North Carolina, I'd often have to drive to the next town over or state to receive services from a free or community clinic. With traffic, that's easily a three hour round trip ride. Very seldom was I able to go with a partner or friend to get tested–that meant carrying the mental stress of how my life would change if I became positive with me to each appointment. I'd receive some form of relief when my results came back negative but pissed at the time I managed to catch a bacteria infection, NGU and chlamydia from playing around.

As a bisexual/pansexual black male, I catch a lot of shit because of my attraction and desire to have sex with men *and* women. Straight women who find out my preference only want me around if they can *honey, boo, chile,* and *girl* with me. And I have never been that nigga. Gay men, especially the black ones, insist that my sexuality is a phase. I get more shit about liking men and women from them than I do anyone else. And the straight black men—some only want me around so they can find out who I fucked so they can mark the women as tainted. Others treat me like I'm diseased or if I have eyes for them. Never mind the fact that these motherfuckers here be the main ones spreading one STI to another amongst their homeboys because they shared the same pussy or got head from the same chick. And the other shenanigans I won't name cause I'm not no snitch.

Like most black men, I avoided the hospital and doctors because I couldn't afford to go—and I didn't want to hear "this was wrong with me" or "that was wrong with me." I think what I feared the most was going to get on PrEP and then finding out that I was indeed positive. When my health would fail–I had no choice but to face it because I'd end up disclosing the "possibility" which prolonged the treatment I needed for whatever it was that brought (FORCED!) me to go to the hospital from the jump.

> As much as I write about male/male/female romances under this literary brand, I would be irresponsible not to promote the use of PrEP (pre-exposure prophylaxis). Using PrEP, while also practicing responsible sexual habits, prevents the possibility of transmitting HIV from vaginal, anal and oral encounters. As a safe sex advocate and ally, I will continue to practice what

> I preach. The pic above is from my prescription I just received and I will be taking my first dose tomorrow. I will be documenting this journey for an upcoming book I have with a media personality.

That's what I posted on my social media accounts when I finally got on PrEP. After reading up and researching, talking to friends and acquaintances who all were on Truvada, I felt I had learned everything I needed to know and was ready to join the others who were "on PrEP." I answered one of the apps on one of the hookup sites and after talking with the nurse, I was alarmed and surprised when they put me on Descovy.

Um, this wasn't what I researched. What was wrong with me that I had to get on Descovy and not Truvada? Nothing against the manufacturers of either medication, but I was adverse to change. It was like being the only one who got the Johnson & Johnson Covid vaccine when everyone else in the family was on Pfizer. I gained more knowledge and considered my own health situation and accepted that my PrEP medication would be handled differently. I decided the possible side effects of diarrhea, nausea, headache, upset stomach were similar to what every other medication advertised on television. I also was happy to learn that I could create children using my own sperm again if I should so choose.

I did not experience those side effects but that doesn't mean that you won't. I'm just happy that I was able to do what was right for me and encourage others to take that step and get on the medication so that one day, HIV would not have the same devastating effects it did in my youth.

PART TWO - EXPLOITATION

THINKING WITH MY DICK

(THE RATING SYSTEM)

I'm sure for the guys who will admit privately, and publicly to having encounters with me, they will want to know how they stacked up against their competition. Part of the reason some of you are reading this is to find out the scoop so why not get into it?

My rating system is not the "be-all, end-all" as I recognize that sexual encounters are personal in nature. What I like and want in an escort may not be what you like and want for services. And that is okay. I'm not here to tell you that you have to like what I like and I'm not guaranteeing that you will have a good time with someone just because I did.

Or that a model who didn't perform for me won't perform for you.

Keep in mind that when it comes to encounters, I am the bottom. Most guys tend to charge more to let you top them. Let's not confuse this with a personal preference. When I'm in relationships or with people whom I can regularly have sexual encounters with–I get plenty of ass. As I've said many times before, my dick works very well. I like to get my dick sucked. I like when my dick is tugged and stroked while my nipples are being licked.

While some people would say I have a type, I'm far from a colorist. When I look in the mirror, I recognize that most people would say at best I have a medium complexion. I recognize the difference between me and Idris Elba or Lance Goss, whom I would define as a handsome, dark-skinned men. I think those who would argue that they, Romance, Too Tough, Xaddy Corvinus and I have the same skin complexion would be making a false statement.

When giving stats, I chose to use the following:

1. Those who stated their stats on Twitter, Instagram, their modeling site, other social media platforms or private messages to me were considered first. That's usually where I start when I select performers I want to have an encounter with. I'm giving the benefit of the doubt to the model when he says he's "6'1." And I'm trusting models to be honest

about their dick sizes. Most of them aren't in a position to lie because their work speaks for themselves.

2. On rare occasions, I've considered sites from recognized publications as primary sources —which I've cited to validate my findings.

Some of the dates or time frames for the encounters are approximations. I can verify those by significant life events, bank statements or communications that I have on file. The number of encounters represents the number of times I've paid for the encounters. The cost of the encounter may be a price or a range depending on my relationship with the model.

Performance level is a sliding scale and in part is based on the following factors:

- Was the model able to perform as promised?
- Did I get the positions requested or promised?
- If the model finishes the job.
- Was I satisfied?

For this exercise, safety is not considered whether or not we wore a condom. I always encourage wearing condoms with me because of my status, and I'm aware that many models may have more than one performance in a small time frame. I commend models who are on PrEP or take responsibility for staying undetectable. As I have chosen to publicly share my status, others may not and I won't violate

HIPPA by sharing someone's status—even if they have confirmed it publicly. Safety for me considers the following:
- Did the model attempt to perform as promised?
- Did the model steal money and or other items during our encounter?
- Did the model threaten physical, verbal or emotional harm?

I have made many attempts and given several models who stole from me or failed to perform services plenty of chances to return funds or make things right with me. Those who did were spared--the rest need to return my money or items.

ADA Friendly is not an endorsement from the Americans with Disabilities Act as I understand that is a law. Some of us in the community use it to define if a person or place is apt to follow the laws and provide us with the services required. Also, us saying ADA Friendly is not a guarantee they will work with someone of a different disability. ADA Friendly, for me, implies was the model considerate of my personal needs. Did they help me with tasks they were told in advance I could or could not do? Were they willing to go the extra mile? I know I can be "a handful" to deal with but, I'm paying for this service and some care needs are part of the service. Anything extra is paid extra and I've been known to tip generously.

Would I recommend to others is straight-forward. Anyone who presents a safety hazard for me and the community will not be recommended.

I know that I'm risking a lot by putting this book together, going on record with encounters and sharing my experience. Maybe I will inspire someone to speak up, and share their experiences. Perhaps some of the bad actors will be shunned out of the industry so that we can continue to support sex work. We can't have a valid industry if one or two bad apples continue to spoil the bunch.

My stats are as follows:

<u>Stats:</u>
Height: 5'6"
Weight: 165 lbs
Dick Size: 8.5 inchesRole: Verse Bottom – Bottom for most paid encounters

Now that I told most of my business, let's get down to what you came for. Who have I fucked? What do I think? Would I recommend?

Let's play ball.

FULL DISCLOSURE

Stats
Height: 6'0"
Weight: 195 lbs
Dick Size: 10.5 inches
Approx. Dates or Time Frames of Encounter:
Number of Encounters: 2
Cost of Encounter: $250/each
Performance Level: 10/10
Is the Escort Safe: Yes
ADA Friendly: Yes
Would I Recommend to Others: Yes

Card Bio: Arguably one of the most versatile (not with men) adult performers to ever grace the planet, Full Disclosure's brand has crossed over to mainstream appeal. His work with female-to-male, trannies and cisgendered women have not gone unnoticed and his ability to give top (especially with men) performances every time has made him a household name. His viral social media clips keep him booked and busy and studios wishing they can lock this head-strung performer down for a flick. His business acumen rivals his onscreen performance, being one of the most successful black (or period) adult performers, male or female. Full Disclosure has perfected a blueprint only matched by few. The best part is that while very little is known about his personal life (other than what he himself has shared), his private life is probably the best kept secret.

The Story:

I have a "love him"/"fuck him" relationship with Full Disclosure.

Look–I don't *hate* Full Disclosure–actually I wish our relationship was a lot better than it is. I hate the shit he has done to me afterward. The pretending he's perfect when he's no saint, the lying and disrespecting my name in public, the working with my enemies for his benefit. I hate all the shit because I always thought he was better than that. I, like many of his fans, watched him build an empire out of this sex work shit. Watched as he put others on and taught others how to *really* get this money. I mean, it's like he's got so fuckin' much but he won't be content until he takes mine, too.

Fuckin' greedy man.

I feel like (no, Cedric feels like) we both do dumb shit to keep each other at each other's throats. We aren't willing to sit down and have the communication we desperately need and the mutuals who know about us and the encounters have worked endlessly to keep us apart.

To a degree, my encounters with him are the bane of my existence. I enjoyed them and of all of the escorts I've been with, he was the best.

There, I said it. Full Disclosure was the best I ever had. A whole fuckin' Drake song.

If you're in this lifestyle, you know hookups are the name of the game. We all got that one (or two) hookup that blew our mind, body and spirit. In the bedroom, this person had the ability to open us up and abandon all of our inhibitions. We love the way they made our body feel and the moments with the person were good–but as human beings, these motherfuckers be trash.

I'm not saying Full Disclosure is trash but a few of the guys who thought they were close, were.

So the million dollar question: why didn't I name Full Disclosure in *Don't Get F+cked Up* and why was he referred to as *Full Disclosure?* Even though some of you who've read this book know who I'm talking about, why won't I name him now?

When we got together to draft and outline what would be included in my memoir, Cedric and I had long discussions on what the storyline would be and how people would be portrayed. Initially, *Piece of Ass* was going to be a separate segment in *Don't Get F+cked Up* where I opened up about sexuality, being a John and dished the dirt.

In writing *Don't Get F+cked Up*, Cedric and I read several biographies from JaRule's *Unruly*, to Eldridge Cleaver's *Soul on Ice* to Hitler's *Mein Kempf* (that was all Cedric–I wouldn't touch that book with a ten-foot pole). We paid particular attention to recently published biographies published after 2017 and we noticed a trend. Many authors and celebrities were acknowledging their recollections as their version of the events and for legal reasons, we state that we may "have altered and changed certain events and names to protect the privacy of certain individuals and organizations. The recollections in this story are Tony's version of the events that have taken place." I'm familiar with the scandal caused by James Frey the author of *A Million Little Pieces* in which it is alleged that most of the book is fiction and not the groundbreaking memoir that changed millions of lives.

Even if we know the events are true, no author takes the risk with the liability and today publishers and distributors can't and won't be willing to face the litigation. It's expensive for all parties involved. With that said, a uniform decision was made to not name any of the escorts who were referenced in the book except for Mike, whom I still have a good relationship with. Also, Mike is not a known porn star or OnlyFans/Freak Twitter content creator. As far as y'all know, Mike with no last name and some descriptions that could fit more than one person, could be anybody.

Another reason I'm acknowledging Full Disclosure is who you think it is as well as admitting that some of you correctly guessed the identities of The Apprentice and SupHomie is because before the publication of this book, it was outed that I had an encounter with Full Disclosure. The drama starters made unsubstantiated allegations as to what I put in the book and what I didn't put in the book. He'd done interviews and had conversations with my frienemies stating that our encounters didn't happen which pissed me off because if you took my money and we had sex more than once, why lie?

I hate that shit.

Let me address the drama starters first none of them had read the book when they put the information out there. Cedric and James were doing final edits because Bethany was on our asses about meeting the deadline. Aside from that—no one had seen the book. Full Disclosure, Aye Papi (whose identity I will not reveal), SupHomie, Too Tough, The Apprentice and a few others were aware that I was working on a book. Most of them were told that *Don't Get F+cked Up* would be autobiographical. In the grand scheme of things, me paying well-known escorts and adult content creators for sex is a small part of my life.

The symptoms from my cerebral palsy and herpes take up quite a bit of my time. Remember, I'm in a wheelchair and I discussed in great detail what it takes to maintain a chair. I've spent most of my life in academia pursuing two bachelors and two masters' degrees—in addition to mentoring and advising quite a few organizations. Most people know or heard of me from interacting with the cast of *Level Up* or *Dreamless Reality*—in other groups and chats where drama and socialites intersect. I'm working to build my clientele as a licensed therapist.

Sex—so little of my time.

What I learned and came to realize in writing *Don't Get F+cked Up* is that these escorts don't appreciate their customers. Most of these guys want to come over, get paid, do minimum work and leave—leaving us unsatisfied and feeling cheated during our encounters. Hence the reason why I'm rating everyone to begin with.

So how much of what I shared in *Don't Get F+cked Up* about my encounter with Full Disclosure is true and how much is make believe? For dramatization purposes, the story shared in *Don't Get F+cked Up* was based on the second encounter and elements of the first encounter were added to enhance the story. All of the elements in the story happened—the tone of the conversation surrounding not being able to check out of my dorm is real.

As Cedric explained to me—biographical books are adapted just like movies and music. So let's consider if I were to have a movie made based on *Don't Get Fucked Up*. Every detail is not going to be dramatized on screen. As books are pushed by words, descriptions that create visualizations and memorable expressions—movies are pushed by dialogue, visuals and to an extent, the people attached to the film. If you thought Cedric and I created dialogue for the book, imagine the amount of work Cedric or another script writer would have to come up with to give you enough dialogue for a ninety minute to two hour movie. It's not like we could read the book word for word—when I get a chance to do that for an audiobook, it's anticipated that my audiobook would be at least eight hours long based on word count. If I did a television show like *Wu-Tang: An American Hip Hop Story*—then each chapter could possibly get its own twenty-three to forty-five minute episode. Certain details that were left out could be expanded and new, fresh dialogue could be written to give characters based on people I know something to talk about.

I was first introduced to Full Disclosure closer to the beginning of his career. He was an up and coming adult entertainer. His locks were just starting, probably two inches long at most. Think J. Cole during the *4 Your Eyez Only* era, but a little shorter. He was dancing for strip clubs up and down the east coast and word was spreading about the videos he had started to make. I had seen a few of his videos and was impressed.

Full Disclosure had the body of an Olympic track star. With his six foot three, one hundred and seventy pounds, he was my definition of edible chocolate. His face had chiseled features that gave hints to Native American ancestry blended with his Caribbean roots. He had no visible tats and he dressed in the latest hip-hop fashions.

His dick was definitely long enough to compete with a Subway foot long.

Our first encounter cost me $250 and was worth every penny. I discovered mobility I had forgotten I had. He had started the process of locking his hair and the promade he used smelled sweet like cotton candy. The scent lingered on my bed sheets a few days after our encounter and helped me bust a few nuts afterward. I had the pleasure of verifying his measurement before we began our session.

"I can't believe it's so big." I didn't mean to come off like a stereotypical blonde bitch but it's true. Everyone talks about ten-inch this, ten-inch that, but Full Disclosure made ten inches look small. Even though this was our second encounter, I still couldn't believe what I was holding in person.

"Not only is it big, it works," he bragged as he wrapped my hand around his meat.

I smirked because I knew that was true.

Up until that point, most of the guys I'd had were eight or nine inches. They were closer to my size and they definitely knew how to work what they had. It was just what Full Disclosure packed in his pants or what he could do with it—it was how he used his whole body to bring the full experience.

Full Disclosure picked me up and turned me upside down. I played the guessing game with how many licks it would take to get it down my throat. He played how many licks it would take to tease my prostate. As many times as he made my body shake, it encouraged me to ensure the tip of his erection hit the back of my throat.

I was surprised that I was able to maintain my balance and focus on the task at hand. After a few more minutes of pleasure, he slowly lifted my body all the way up. He cupped my ass like he was grabbing cantaloupe. "I'm gonna lower you all the way down my dick."

Hell yeah I was nervous. I wasn't on my hands and knees so I couldn't run. "You can grip my arms or rest your hands around my neck," he encouraged as he lowered me on his pole. I was surprised that I was able to get down quite a bit of his length. I locked eyes with him, which was a mistake on my part. Full Disclosure continued to make sure the tip of his dick broke through my second hole. I screamed and shouted like I enjoyed the best ride at the theme park.

If that wasn't enough, he put me on all fours and pounded me out. I see why he started going by the name that's made him most famous. The stroke was something serious and a weaker bottom would fall or run. I'd heard of encounters he's had with others where they tapped out. I was determined not to be one.

I came multiple times, once without touching myself. I didn't think that was possible. After he dropped his load, we both rested on the bed for a minute. It felt good laying next to him, even if just for a few seconds. I didn't get attached to the feeling because I knew I was going to have to get up and face reality. The money I owed for this encounter already left my account and I was contemplating giving him a tip.

In the second encounter, the sexual experience was unique and just as good and once it was over, that's when the drama started.

"Is the dude gonna be at the front desk so I can get my ID back?" Full Disclosure asked as he adjusted his oversized Sean Jean fit.

"Yeah, we shouldn't have a problem," I answered as I looked at the clock. We were past the curfew but no one had ever had a problem with their guest leaving. Unlike many of my peers, I typically checked my guests in and most of the attendants didn't mind if I went over my time.

I worked quickly to get myself dressed and in the chair so I could go with him and we could hang for a while before he left. I knew I wanted another encounter and I hoped to be able to set that up.

Once we left my room, rolled behind to get to the building where he had checked in at. Full Disclosure walked very fast and was hard to keep up with, even with my motorized chair.

We arrived at the building and the attendant wasn't at the desk.

"I don't have all day," Full Disclosure grew impatient as he banged on the desk. I pulled out my phone so I could call one of the attendants who could get his ID and check him out.

"Bruh, I'm not trying to be trapped here with you," Full Disclosure directed his anger at me. "I need to get the fuck out of here because I got someplace to be." His tone got more aggressive with me.

Trapped. That word broke me out of the illusion that there would be a third encounter or that he enjoyed himself with me. Honestly, I wanted to cry but I couldn't. I would not show him weakness.

I couldn't get no one on the phone, which was unusual because I didn't see that they had called when he stayed past our dorm curfew. Usually, the attendants would call or make an announcement on the intercom for our guests to come down. Sometimes, I avoided that fate because it was assumed that my visitors were helping me get ready to leave.

"Yo!" Full Disclosure got more agitated. "You said I'd be able to sign out quickly."

"I don't know, this is not my fault." I defended myself. "They knew you were up here with me so I don't know what's going on."

Full Disclosure was pissing me off. The last thing I wanted was to beg him to stay with me. After an hour of listening to him rant and rave, the attendant came to the office and signed him out. To this day, Full Disclosure acts like I orchestrated this whole event. I already paid this man for good sex, and even though he irritates the fuck out of me, I'm not going to deny we had good sex. But I'm sick of these motherfuckers feeling like they can talk to me any kind of way and treat me with malice. I watched him storm off after getting his ID and the attendant apologized to me.

"It's okay," I told him. I made a note to myself that I would never let a trick treat me like this again. What should have been an enjoyable occasion turned into a nightmare I still re-live from time to time.

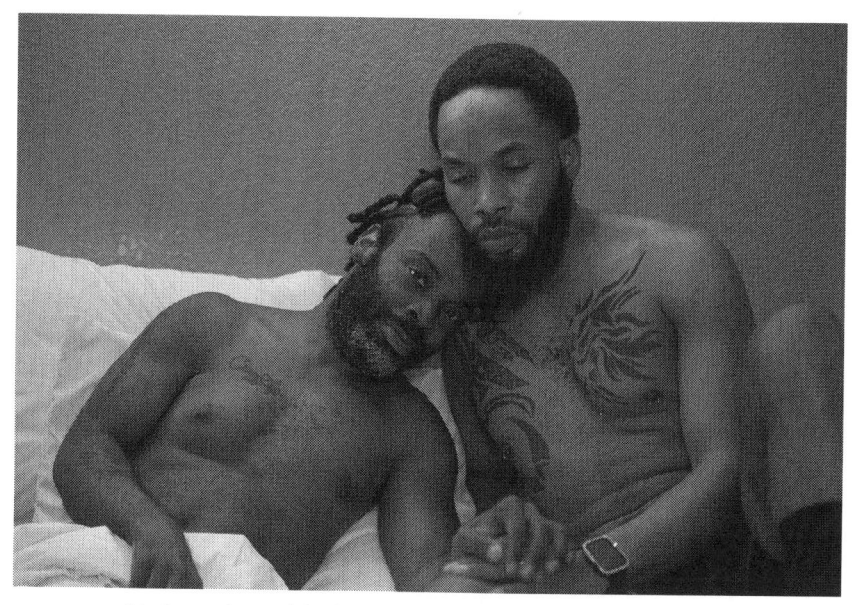

Nyjewel and I during a photoshoot.

AYE PAPI

<u>Stats</u>
Height: 6'0"
Weight: 195 lbs
Dick Size: 11.5 inches
Approx. Dates or Time Frames of Encounter: Since 2015
Number of Encounters: Several and counting.
Cost of Encounter: Varies based on encounter
Performance Level: 9.5/10
Is the Escort Safe: Yes
ADA Friendly: One of the best.
Would I Recommend to Others: Hell yes!!!

<u>Card Bio:</u> Doesn't need one.

I'm allowed to have secrets and the identity of Aye Papi will be one of them. None of you whom have speculated on his identity have been right so far. Now if he comes out and says something, then okay. But I seriously doubt he will.

PIECE OF ASS

The Story:

In *Don't Get F+cked Up*, I described my relationship with Aye Papi as a teenage love affair. In fact, I almost named the chapter after one of my favorite Alicia Keys songs.

One thing Karine Steffans taught me when reading her book, *Confessions of a Video Vixen*, is that it is okay to keep secrets (not an irony). Don't get it twisted, I belong to a Greek-Lettered Organization and I know what discretion is, but as a personality, I'm not obligated to share every little detail with the public. So I'm gonna keep y'all guessing about Aye Papi.

I will say that those in my era will recognize him as he's made more than one memorable video. Aye Papi is my ideal man physically–tall, the color of a perfect brew of French Vanilla coffee. Slender, basketball center framed. Aye Papi could have easily been a model for a major fashion brand, but I fear he had too much swagger for the white men. He's not a "yes man" and I even had a few run-ins with his notorious temper. But I meant what I said about his eleven and a half inches of meat playing a role in how he got his name. He was a thug's, thug–street personality, hood mentality. Kelly and them were singing about my man in "Soldier" while getting T. I. and Lil' Wayne pretending to be him. Someone said that French Montana sold "thug on a sex appeal"–so did Aye Papi.

I viewed Aye Papi as my lover, even though I did pay for his services. Unlike some of the other escorts I worked with, there was a "relationship" aspect to our situation. Unlike many men, Aye Papi did help take care of me. He would wash my body, help me get into my chair, clean my room and didn't mind being seen with me in public. I'm sure those who saw me with him who were in the lifestyle would know who he is because we did walk/roll around campus or seen eating together in public frequently. I did meet his family and got to hang with him socially. If it weren't for the fact that I was paying him, Aye Papi could have easily been a boyfriend.

Oh how the girls would gag if I was rolling next to him as we walked through campus, ate at fine restaurants, chilled at social events, all while saying "that's my man." Think these bitches talk about me, they couldn't take it if we were able to do that.

In the same breath that I'd want to brag and boast about landing Aye Papi, my self esteem fell with every dollar I paid him. Every touch felt so real, but when it was over. When he put on his boxers, sagged his sweat pants just right, grabbed his shit and left my room or wherever we were fucking at–I felt my spirit fall to the floor.

Once he penetrated my walls, made me scream and shout, feel human for a minute, I'd be left thinking this is a nightmare once it was all over with. I'd hustle for every nickel and dime to spend some time with my "boyfriend."

Why did it have to be like this?

In my mind, I was crazier than Heather Headley because all I wanted was to spend more time with him. With Aye Papi, I felt like the clocks stopped ticking as I cherished our moments together.

Aye Papi was a boyfriend but he wasn't perfect–I knew how to bring the monster out of him. I wouldn't say he was physically abusive toward me, but he was possessive in other ways. To be honest, he'd kicked The Apprentice's ass if he knew I spent some time with him. Aye Papi wanted me to be his only trick–but it was okay for him to fuck all these niggas and bitches on film and behind closed doors.

***

I rolled myself into a conference room on the third floor. The person who was assisting me in navigating to the room was a bit frustrated because "they didn't think they were gonna have to do that much work."

Bitch!

I thought I was gonna get whiplash from how fast I turned my head. The audacity and gall to say that aloud behooves me. Especially since I was paying them outta pocket for this service. I would have wrapped this person's neck around the handle of my chair if I hadn't come here to do battle. I needed to save my energy. But this is an example of the slick ass comments from escorts and "regular people" alike.

"You are being compensated," I reminded this person as nicely as I could as I navigated my chair around to my side of the conference table. I watched as my nemesis and his party rolled in. He scrunched his nose and mumbled something under his breath about it smelling like "stale overcooked onions" and the administrative party around him trying to hide a chuckle.

I refrained from replying with my middle finger.

The bad thing about going to the HBCU was that it was not accessible to people with special needs. There were no ramps or rollaways that would make traveling across the university easy. The elevators were out of order, many were old and outdated and in desperate need of repairs. Sometimes the working elevators were not accessible even though it was known that I would need access so that I could get to classes that were often on the second and third floors. I felt at times that I was intentionally being barred from moving around the campus freely. If they could confine me, they could make me quit. I know that's what some people wanted and why I put up with this abuse is what baffles me the most. This is classic Stockholm syndrome because even as I dictate this, I want nothing but the best for the university, the staff and its students. I still make myself available for any and all, regardless of fraternal or academic affiliation. While I will not say that I believe that the university itself had these views, I wouldn't put it past certain figures for doing little things here or there to get their point across.

This is the side of my life that many people would like to push out of the way and pretend like it doesn't happen. Or that my need to be transported by wheelchair is an inconvenience *to them*. There were times when I was treated like my existence was a burden they carried the weight of. The reality is, I wake up with my burden every day. I did not ask to be born with cerebral palsy. I did not ask to not be able to walk like "most" people or to be punished as if I committed a crime against humanity.

On the same day that I was meeting Aye Papi, I was fighting allegations that I had cheated on my project. The professor, Dr. Foundation, wanted me academically dismissed from the program and expelled from the university. He and I never got along. However, he had influence in the direction of the program I was pursuing and the university often acquiesced to his demands to make him happy and to keep him on board.

One of the things that I appreciated about Aye Papi that I talked about in *Don't Get F+cked Up*, there was a friendship to our situation. I'm not gonna sit here and say I talk to him for two or three hours at a time and he's always doing me favors and we were best friends. However, out of all of the escorts aside from SupHomie, whom I'll talk about later, Aye Papi was the closest thing I would have to a boyfriend. I knew a lot of things about his life that I'm not going to share in this book that the average porn, viewer, or person in our LGBTQ space wouldn't know. Equally, he knew mine. When I was in his presence, whether we were on the campus or off, he never let anyone disrespect me because of my condition. I always had a friend in him, even if our sexual relationship was contractual.

"Slobbers does not deserve to be among us!" Dr. Foundation shouted and shook as he closed his argument. I hated that he'd gone out of his way to create a nickname for me that he reveled in insulting me in his classroom—what's worse was that he was so comfortable with his disrespect, that he'd openly call me disparaging names in front of his colleagues at this HBCU. Legally, I can't discuss too much about the case surrounding this and other allegations pertaining to this issue, but I can say that of all the people who tried to bully me and make me feel unwelcome, Dr. Foundation was the worst.

I leaned in to my representative, who I would later learn had a conflicting relationship with the university, "ask him about the lack of accommodations I needed for my project."

"I don't think we should do that Tony," he quickly moved away from me and dismissed my concern.

Here I was again, in a fight where I was outnumbered seven to one. Getting jumped as I'm fighting for my life despite being the one with the handicaps and disadvantages. Would've thought I was Goliath the way they ganged up on me.

Dr. Foundation glared at me as he attempted to make his five foot six, two hundred and fifty pound frame seem imposing. His skin glistened as if he'd been placed in the spotlight. His voice projected as if the conference room were a Broadway stage—the people in the nosebleed section of the theater would've heard him. "I don't even know why we're here. It's clear that the boy cheated. He can't write worth a damn. He looks like a rejected tattered doll from the *Child's Play* movie and he talks like he's chewing on marshmallows and lead."

This was tame compared to the curse words and harsh insults he'd direct toward me from the comfort of the classroom and in front of my peers. Some who would laugh with him. Those who would challenge the mistreatment would find themselves targeted by him and his friends.

"The insults aren't necessary," I defended myself when I wanted to retaliate.

"You're not to speak directly to him." My representative warned me.

"But he can say whatever he wants to me?!" I tried my best not to curse this man out because I'm used to it being me against the world everywhere I go. I was tired of always taking the high road when these motherfuckers roll me through the mud and fling shit at me from up high. I was equally impatient with always being set up with the most incompetent people who do not have my best interest at heart, care about my well-being and just overall assholes to me. I needed this Judas who was supposed to be helping me to do his job so that I could pursue next steps if I chose.

"Tony, you need to be professional." I was admonished by the "leader" in the room.

"So should he." I returned this candy Whopper-shaped head motherfucker's glare. I never understood how a world-renown national best selling author, who stayed on somebody's television show, felt intimidated about me. This asshole was tenured at the university, again, he has everything. Money, power, respect, and he is still not happy.

He can't be if he's worried about me.

Aye Papi mentioned that Dr. Foundation gave him an attitude when he was waiting for me outside of class one day. Every time I hung out with Aye Papi, it wasn't just for sex or companionship. We'd talk about our personal lives. I explained to him why I liked studying people and how I thought I could help make the world a better place.

What pisses me off about my interactions with Dr. Foundation is that his behavior toward myself and others with mental and physical disabilities is condoned. Everyone with leverage knows that he is a discriminatory, dick sucking, open closeted-door prick. Yet, no one besides me is bold enough to challenge him on his actions. When I first met him I was humbled and had aspirations of being mentored by him. Nowadays if I had to choose between saving his life or resurrecting a mass murderer, well let the reign of terror begin.

"He probably wants to suck my dick," Aye Papi brought me back to focus on this encounter. I laughed as I could picture Aye Papi roughly grabbing Dr. Foundation's head and guiding up and down his man stick.

"I think he's mad that I'm getting fucked by you tonight." I smirked.

I had one-upped Dr. Foundation and every gatekeeping prick like him. I wondered how many other escorts I fucked that were out of reach for him. He had more money, yet *I* kept getting the men.

Damn.

"They still think that you copied that guy's paper?" Aye Papi questioned as he followed me rolling out of the building.

"Yeah." I was irritated but I didn't want that bullshit meeting where they tried to get me to "confess" to cheating to get to me.

"I remember you helping that dude and another group of people in the library a few weeks ago."

I remembered sucking his dick in the bathroom afterward and then him fucking me in the suite I shared with three other guys. Too bad I didn't have the money to repeat that situation because I sure could use a beating now.

"So where do we go from here?"

We? I liked how it seemed like I was getting closer to "boyfriend" status. Aye Papi was concerned for my well-being and that was one of the reasons I sometimes got my role as a John confused with being "boyfriend." Most of the escorts I dealt with wouldn't give two fucks whether I took my next breath, as long as they got my last dollar they were good. But Aye Papi was more than that. Even when we weren't having sex and we had conversations, he genuinely seemed to be concerned about my mental and physical health. To the point that I'd probably have to credit him with some of the physical abilities I had because sex with him definitely forced me to do my therapeutic exercises.

"Well, it would be good if I could find a *real* lawyer so I wouldn't feel like I was getting played all the damn time." I vented as I continued to roll across campus.

"How much would one cost?" He asked as he moved the lever on my chair forward. I caught a few glances from some of the campus gays that I knew recognized him. I knew they couldn't take that I was with him. Chile. But they knew not to confront me about it. That's one thing I can say about the gays at the University, they didn't appear to be as messy as some of the gays in the perimeter were in general. To be honest, they probably wouldn't believe that I was paying him for his service if I told them.

"$10,000 I don't have." I lamented as we finally got to the crosswalk. We looked both ways before we crossed the street. At this time in my life all I wanted was to proceed forward so that I could practice therapy in Georgia. I didn't want to have to move back home, because I knew that if I had to go back to St. Louis, there was a pretty good chance I would never make it back to Atlanta. Living in Atlanta has given me full freedom. I got to choose when I got up, how late I stayed out, who I hung around, and I didn't have to worry about being in a house or of adults and kids trying to survive. It's love my family, but I'm a young man with a hungry appetite for sex. Gay sex. And I need space and opportunity to explore this side of me. Try to live life without as much attention brought to my physical limitations as possible.

That's probably why sex was so important to me and why I put up with paying these escorts to begin with. In Atlanta, the dating pool for men with my ideal specs were much larger. And even if I just wanted to hook up, I have more opportunities to do it here.

With Aye Papi, I spent so much time living life. The good thing was that in this interim, I had contributed to *The Black Man's Guide to Graduate School* in which I and five other authors offered tips and guidance for other black men interested in going to graduate school. A few years later, I would begin the draft for *Don't Get F+cked Up* while engaging in drama with the social media girlies.

Even with all this drama, one of the things I remember about Aye Papi the most is that with him I enjoyed freedom. I was the most mobile, I got to be seen and socialized, and I have to say he's one of the very few I've dealt with who can hold an intelligent conversation. Engagement with him validated everything I knew to be true about myself. It reminded me of the core reasons in which I chose to become a mental health professional. My belief in people and their ability to transition from their current situation mirrors the fight I have with my own physical limitations every day. I enjoy being able to show that despite what you can see on the outside, that I have a wealth of knowledge to share, and if you entertained a decent conversation with me any of the time, I could contribute to a solution to your problems.

What I appreciated with Aye Papi was that everything wasn't "just sex" with him—even if it was supposed to be.

DOIN' IT

(ROLLON REBEL INTERLUDE A PRETTY PRIVILEGE DISS TRACK)

I'm taking a break from talking about fucking these niggas. I feel like I need to remind the readers that I'm not here to tell you about every famous ballroom performer, porn star, content creator, or web series actor I've ever slept with. I already know from when the last book came out that there's gonna be some issues because I dare to admit that I got some "famous" dick. And I use the word "famous" very fucking loosely. As I discussed in the last book, and even parts of this one, I do have a type. Tall, light skin, long hair, light brown eyes, built like a basketball player—specifically a point guard. Can pull off the edgy, street guy look.

I was saying ten inches or bigger before Left Eye was, don't get mad. I'm just good at being bad.

And while I have a type, I have not been exclusively honoring my preference. I feature all types of guys.

Full Disclosure fucked me multiple times in the two encounters I paid for and he was the best (unfortunately) to date and he doesn't fit most of my preferences, so how do I explain that?

Some guys were left out not because I want it balanced, but because they weren't that great. I should share that many of your faves can't keep a hard dick—that's why they're scammers. Watch the videos carefully. If you can't see an angle of the hard dick penetrating an ass, that's a good sign the content creators are faking it.

The truth is BL Rhames' Sims character can keep it harder than you do.

Cedric made me leave some of y'all out so I wouldn't air y'all out, cause if it were up to me, I'd blast a lot of you. But then, why give these motherfuckers promotion? Let's think about things for a minute. A lot of the guys who I've had conflicts with were selected to be on someone else's platform, right? They come on various shows, get their fifteen minutes of fame, and aside from a few followers on social media, very few of them have done anything else. Yeah, a few of them have tried adult content platforms, but where has that left them? How many of these people who feel like they are A-list celebrities have really taken this platform and built a viable, financially-sound brand that brings them revenue they actually can live off of?

Some of these guys who were "it" in 2020 can't be found now. I'm not gonna name names, but where are they? Before the pot calls the kettle black one could say the same thing about me. A lot of y'all met me through trying to support social media personalities I liked, and thought I could bond with. Many of you witnessed me coming to the aid and defense of certain content creators while trying to make others who, I thought were just a little flawed, see the error in their ways. I stay on Facebook and Twitter beefing with some people. That's not my goal in life, to stay in beefs, but people feel comfortable picking on me but I'm gonna always defend myself.

Considering how some of these same people have shown their head, shoulders, knees and toes, and all of their two thousand body parts on a worn Lever 2000 soap bar, what do they have to show for? I thought the investigation of whether or not I had a license to practice therapy in Missouri and Georgia was cute. Imagine the embarrassment that came about when you found out it was true. Thinking of the humiliation when you realize, "oh, he's actually been a licensed therapist for almost ten years." Or, "he's been advocating for disabled people for all his life." I have three undergraduate and graduate degrees, and you have none, sir. That doesn't make me better than you, but that does pose the question of why I have ambition, and you have access to resources and have none?

I told y'all when I first got on these platforms in 2017 that I was working on a book and getting my ideas together. Never mind the fact that I had already co-authored one book at this point. I had already drafted a version of *Don't*

Get F+cked Up that some of my naysayers and other critics were privy to on various private social media groups. If I ever get *that* version of the book back, I could just pay Cedric or someone else to tweak it, and release it as another book, since it was significantly different from what I ended up publishing a few years ago.

Piece of Ass makes book number three and my documentary will establish my platform independently of the very people who rely on other peoples platforms to talk shit about me. And another thing, with the exception of my first book, I own the content to two books and my documentary outright. As technology gets better, I'll be able to decide if, when, and how to release my content to new platforms. I'll decide what paywalls my content will be behind and how it will be paid for. Unlike these other knuckleheads, I am in control of my image and my platform. They are dependent on someone else's stability or interest in which to build theirs.

So run that back about how you're doing better than me again?

Those nudes you leaked, I actually *own* those pictures and I could sue at any time. This is not about me making threats in my own book. This is me stating facts. Let's be honest readers, how many of these guys have you seen me in beef with who still have moderately successful platforms independent of the web series or the adult content creation sites they are mainly associated with? I could name two, but they wouldn't need me to further their platforms, and I wouldn't want to.

To The Apprentice's credit, he's been showing people for the last fifteen years how to do it correctly and very few have followed the blueprint he's easily laid before us. I am admitting that he has outright shown a step-by-step guide on how to build your own platform that you own correctly, and most people haven't followed it.

Let the same motherfuckers think they are hot shit because they've allowed you to believe that they got to fuck some of the same Insta/social media "celebrities" I fucked for free. The truth is they've paid just as much, if not more than what I've paid. The hard truth is that these guys had the same problem with each other that I have with them. They won't admit it publicly or if they do, they act like their issue was different than mine. It's the same shit, different day.

So to the people who've only been on one season or two of a respectable *Web Series/Reality Show*, where have you been since your last season? Where is that store *you* said you were opening? Oh, you don't have the money to start it yet. Where is the new webseries you were working on to showcase your "acting" skills? Let me find out you couldn't afford to pay a ghostwriter or two or five to whip something together for you. Maybe the truth is some of the people who you thought were your "friends" who you thought were gonna "write this show for you" decided they weren't going to do it for free once they got started and when they sent you an invoice, you couldn't pay it. Or, the truth is you tried to write the script yourself, realized how difficult writing can be when you're not committed to working on the craft daily, and you put your dream to the side.

You couldn't scam the photographer, and they deleted the footage rather than give it to you. There wasn't enough ass or dick to give out to keep it, boo.

You owe the producer of the album you were working on money for both the beats they put together, and the studio time that you wasted because you weren't prepared to sing a note when you got into the booth. You were too busy talking shit online, or trying to fuck everything in sight to practice for your upcoming show. That's the *real reason* you can't stay booked.

Your ex leaked your nudes. You regret celebrating the way mine were leaked and your feelings are hurt because the ten inches you bragged about having looked more like five inches or no inches. There's nothing wrong with a smaller dick except your stroke game was worse than a pencil struggling to poke through a sponge. Your ass had no jiggle and you weren't clapping cheeks but struggling to stay on the sheets.

The truth is you're better off on the bottom than trying to be somebody's "masculine top." Yet bottoming goes against the image you've been led astray to believe you created for yourself. The guy we fucked said I was a better top than you.

Word on the internet and in the perimeter is that you painted a well-known performer and if he sees you again, you know he's gonna kick your ass.

The paragraph above applies to a few of y'all. One of you owes me a few hundred dollars I paid from keeping your video from leaking—despite how you've treated me.

The karma from the money you stole from my ATM card to get your ass tatted and enhance your deflated BBL is you and your boyfriend having to look over your shoulder because another ex you scammed found you after he "suddenly" got out of jail.

Everyone finally sees how crazy your demented ass really is with your made up family, instability and grave concern that you are better off in some form of institution so that you can be supervised. What made you think he was staying forever?

Dogging me on social media but crying to me for help in texts and private messages—if I were a savage, I'd leak the screenshots and the FaceTime of what should have been a solo flick that turned into a cry for help.

No one's rooting for you slapping the guy in your chair —it was all in your mind.

I could put names to all this shit but why? This interlude was a compromise. And a warning. Leave me the fuck alone. Stop trying to cheat me out of services I paid for. Pay me what you owe—give me what I pay for.

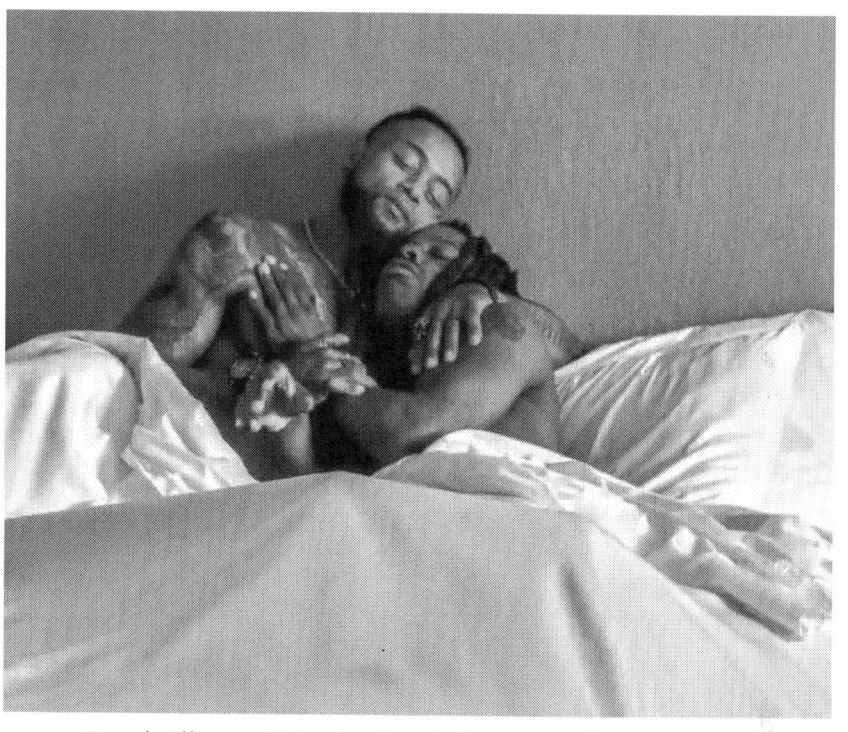

Freakzilla and I in the bed during a photoshoot.

TOO TOUGH

Stats
Height: 6'1"
Weight: 140 lbs
Dick Size: 9.5 inches

Approx. Dates or Timeframes of Encounter: 2018 - My Birthday
Number of Encounters: 1
Cost of Encounter:
Performance Level: 8/10
Is the Escort Safe: Yes
ADA Friendly: Yes
Would I Recommend to Others: Yes-if he's available.

<u>Card Bio:</u> Too Tough benefited from an unconventional background in the adult world. His initial claim to fame was a recurring role on a prominent Ballroom Throwbacks TV (BRTB TV) show before starring in a few webseries for HD Productions. On his social media accounts from that time period, you would mainly see pics of him showing off his body. The rare post would come from the world many other people know him from—the ballroom scene. In those competitions, Too Tough is known for voguing and presenting "masculine realness." While he had a subscription site and the occasional nude/sex scene in a webseries, very few people have videos of him performing solo or partner sex acts.

PIECE OF ASS

The Story:

In 2018, I spent most of my time trying to figure out how I was going to get back to Atlanta. The past few years have not been great for me personally, or professionally. I was still dealing with the fallout from being dismissed from the masters program at the HBCU, and trying to salvage my reputation in the academia world. In addition, my health was on a decline. The herpes flare ups would happen more frequently. My legs got weaker, making it hard to stand even for seconds at a time. While I encouraged others to be strong and fought many battles publicly, privately, I felt like I was losing my fuckin' mind. All this while trying to figure out how to get back into the job market after having to take disability to survive.

On the surface, most people have known me as Tony Rebel and saw me engaging in conflict with some of the participants and various low budget "reality shows" that appeared on YouTube. I'd participate as an audience member, and I give feedback where I felt it was due. But it always seem like somebody wanted to fuck with me because they ain't like what I had to say. They always were threatening to slap me, knock me out of my chair, and just talking regular gay shit to make themselves look better. Never understood why people felt like they had to put someone else down to lift themselves up. I wanted to participate in a couple of reunions, and maybe even be a guest or friend of a show I knew was filming around that time, which made sense because people would finally be able to put a name to a face. I'd finally be able to show my authentic self, and people were seeing that I was who I knew I was.

As I'm always the direct and assertive type, I stayed in conflict. At this time, I was dealing with the beef with another "social media personality" who was promoting and showcasing my leaked nude photos. In the picture, I had laid on my side, facing the wall on the bed. My back was to the photographer. The person taking the picture had done a good job of presenting me in a vulnerable yet artistic state. My imperfect body was exposed and people could see the bruises and scars that came from some of the surgeries I had. I was surprised that people were excited to see me in that way, and if I didn't know better, I'd thought I was on one of the adult videos the people were sneaking to watch on MyVidster, or Pornhub. People critique the way my body looked in, criticize me for not being a tiptop, athletic shape. What these assholes felt to realize that I was completely physically disabled. It's not that I wanted to be an adult star or become known for my body–I didn't expect people to have a reaction to it.

On the inside, a thousand questions ran through my mind because I didn't know how people would react to seeing me this way. I didn't want the picture to become all of who Tony Rebel was. I didn't want this to affect who I was professionally and I didn't want this to be how people were introduced to me. In time, I came to see it as fair game. Not that I'd leak someone's personal nude photo that was sent to me or that I had paid for but I'm out there. Some of them would never be.

As I got past this distraction I began to focus on the real issue at hand. I didn't want to just return to Atlanta to visit or study–I wanted to become a permanent resident and I knew I was going to need steady income in order to deal with the area's growing cost and increasing population. I had a license to practice therapy in Missouri and still saw the occasional client here and there. This was good because I still had residence in Missouri and I could practice with Missouri-based clients anywhere as long as my license was current. I did the work to maintain my licensure by taking continuing education classes so that I can stay current and study. I saw my fight to become a licensed therapist in the State of Georgia as being my ticket to financial and personal freedom. I had started working on the book sporadically and thankfully, Cedric, James, and D. Rashad Battle would take my phone calls and answer questions privately about how to proceed in moving forward with my book. During this time, I was heavily dependent upon my sister and certain extended family members for my personal care and some activities of daily living.

Don't get me wrong, I don't hate the city of St. Louis, but I've always felt that my true home was in the A. I wanted to be in a town where I can openly and freely be me unapologetically. Participate in the social life I had become a custom to while being a student. Be able to show everyone that I had grown up. Many people in my age group and educational status struggled to live independently because of being behind in the job market and the lack of opportunities that steel did not exist for us. Many of my peers would have to learn new trades and change job markets to make ends meet.

They have those options, I did not.

So after dealing with the stress of being in St. Louis another year, and missing my friends, I plotted to get back to Atlanta. I had gotten into a bad car accident a few years prior and any day now, we were waiting on the settlement since the driver of the other vehicle was at fault. In addition, I was appealing my academic dismissal, and dealing with some of the legal ramifications from that.

I wanted it, no I need some dick. It had been over a year since I had been intimate with anyone and during my previous trip to Atlanta. I planned a hook up session with a previous escort that I had dealt with fell through. I wanted to celebrate my birthday in style, and I initially pursued another escort that I have been in contact with who told me they would be in town for my birthday.

When I initially approached Too Tough it wasn't about linking up, while I was getting the writers together, I wanted him to be on the cover of my book. He was on the shorter end of guys I'd deal with but like I said, I didn't want him for that. I wanted Too Tough to be on the book cover because I wanted to showcase someone who had a more contemporary look and feel. He could look tough in the right amount of street clothes but those of us who know, know he can get down for the girls.

I followed him on social media because I was a fan of the work he'd done on various webseries and I thought that he was cool to engage with. I liked the pictures he posted because they were classy–I don't remember him showing print boldly. His Onlyfans he'd later create became a behind-closed-doors extension of what you'd see on the site. We had chatted and talked a few months before we met up on my birthday.

I had just hung out with some of my friends and he agreed to meet me at my room. I was excited because, again, I wasn't expecting anything from him. I liked the idea of meeting him face to face, not just talking with him online. When I saw him, he looked just like the boy in the picture. He sounded masculine, too.

We went to my room and I noticed he seemed very stand-offish and tense. "Do I make you uncomfortable?" I knew the answer was *yes* but I wanted to see if he would admit it. Be a man and tell me the deal–don't you spend all this time talking to me when we're online but now that we're face to face, you got cobwebs in your mouth?

"It's not really something I do," he finally answered. "I'm not a prostitute–I mean, I can be when I want to but I don't always want to."

"Why don't you want to fuck with me?"

"I'm not with you in the chair." He stammered.

"You're not going to fuck me in the chair," I was patient and observed him as I responded.

"It's just," he hesitated. I respect the fact that he was trying not to hurt my feelings. I knew he could be very blunt if he wanted to be. "I don't think I can do this."

"Do you want to leave?" I offered. I could get my money back and just chill–doubt I'd find someone else this late and the day that wasn't going to be an arm and a leg or ready to perform on short notice.

"Yes–no. I mean, it would be wrong to cancel on you on such short notice."

"But I don't want to force you to do something you don't want to do." I got to the point. "I get it that I'm repulsive to some and if that's the thing for you, you can walk out of the door and we can still be cool."

Too Tough stood up and he surprised me by pulling his pants down. "Can we work up to it?"

I looked at his dick and I was surprised he was packing–but the skinny ones usually are. His pubes were neatly trimmed and faint traces of Irish Spring was a pleasant delight. His balls looked full and the perfect cushion to his meaty package. His mushroom tip seemed to rest comfortably between. I wrapped my fingers around it, tickling his veins, following the trail in hopes of awaking the nerves and increasing the blood flow. Once he became erect, I gripped his dick and stroked him slow and steady. I looked at him and I could see him closing his eyes tight. I knew he was pretending that I was someone else. Hurt my feelings and to be honest, I didn't want to continue because it made me reflect on how I'd stooped to this–paying guys for sex. I think he forgot that part of the service was making sure that *I* felt wanted and desired. That *I* got pleasure.

I'd already paid him.

Truthfully, I wanted to stop but hearing "Birthday Sex" blasting so loud from the car pulling up to a room near mine reminded me why I was here. I deserved what Jeremih was singing about. As I went down on him, I started to pretend he was someone else, but that couldn't do it for me. Then I pretended that he was thinking about me but I couldn't stay with that vibe for long. Eventually, I went with the motions until he was ready to mount me.

Then I did the same shit I always do–get on my knees, put my head down and wait for him to give me strokes. As he spread my cheeks to get easier access to my hole, I frowned. I fought back a tear–not of joy but of sorrow as he penetrated me. I went with the motions, kept up with his strokes as I cried through the moans of pleasure.

It's not that Too Tough didn't fuck me right–it's knowing he never wanted to fuck me. That night or any night. I was getting pity sex for my birthday and if I hadn't been so badly beaten and bruised before, this would've been the worst birthday present ever.

He came and I could barely feel the explosion inside me. I'm used to dudes increasing the tempo, feeling their dicks expand, getting a sense of euphoria once thick hot liquid sprayed my insides. With Too Tough, I didn't feel anything.

I wondered if he faked it. I started to push out to see if I could get his nut to drip from my hole to my gooch but then I thought to myself *why bother?* I laid down and turned to watch him get dressed. The body I once admired and complemented was soon covered with the typical branded sweat clothed gear. He said some words I didn't remember. I fought back tears as he left the room. I sat up and grabbed the sheets tighter than Eddie Murphy did in *Boomerang*. Except this time when I threw the toy, I knew I didn't want it to come back.

THE APPRENTICE

Stats
Height: 6'1"
Weight: 187 lbs
Dick Size: 9 inches

Approx. Dates or Timeframes of Encounter:
Number of Encounters: 2

Cost of Encounter: $500/hour
Performance Level: 7 out of 10
Is the Escort Safe: Yes
ADA Friendly: No
Would I Recommend to Others: With Reservation

Card Bio: Respected for his strong business acumen as well as his predominantly top performances, The Apprentice modeled early on for his peers that to have a long-standing career, one must put in high quality work and take ownership of their brand. While The Apprentice started out and was highly known for his boyish looks in his scenes with predominantly black productions like DawgPoundUSA, and Chocolate Drop, he achieved bigger success with the launch of The Apprentice Corporation. Through his brand, he not only controls a respectable number of his memorable photoshoots and scenes, The Apprentice has branched out into music, film and being a spokesperson for branded products.

The Story:

The Apprentice physically fits the bill of my preferred type. But I want so much more than a light skinned man to lay up with at night. It would be nice not to have an argument every time we communicate.

We fucked twice, it was nice and he's worth it for his price. You've seen his dick, I've felt his stroke, it's better than the average poke.

I enjoyed sex with The Apprentice, I don't enjoy the engagement with him or how he treats me as his customer. Like my money isn't good enough or that he's too good to be in my presence. If you feel that way, why do you fuck with me? Why answer my calls? Am I back on your mailing list after I unsubscribed from your services? Your boyfriends get tired of being abused by you so you reach out to me because you have no one to talk down to?

You need my money don't you?

The Apprentice makes me think I have an addiction to abuse. Yeah, when I think about all the bullshit I dealt with and talked about with in *Don't Get F+cked Up*, it makes perfect sense. And I'm guilty because I *allow* this to happen. I *allow* The Apprentice to feel like he's next to God and that he's better than me. I'm just as bad as the other thousands of people who continue to buy into and support his bullshit.

I think I'm attracted to the regular engagement. He's usually nice to me at first. We apologize to one another and we go through the motion of working toward bettering our relationship. We've been doing this for a few years now and when the last book came out, we were on our shit again. By time this book comes out or the documentary (whichever comes first), we'll be back at it.

There are moments when I wish this were different. I deserve better but it's not often that I have better. This back and forth and arguing over whether I'm going to be his John or not and about what happened in the past beats arguing back and forth with them hating ass internet sissies. I'm addicted to this toxic behavior and don't know how to get off this merry-go-round that always produces the same result. Even when I block his sites, delete his number from my phone, this motherfucker always finds a way back. He pops up in a "classic video" or in arguments with people on BIGO and he makes sense sometimes and I compliment him.

Then the cycle starts over again.

After the release of *Don't Get F+cked Up*, he denied having sex with me or taking money and threatened to sue me. How? When I literally have the screenshots where he continuously reminds me that I need to pay to have sex with him, again? How am I having sex with you, again, if I didn't have sex with you the first two times? Put it together Sherlock.

Yet, this is my fault because I *allow* this. I'm guilty of a classic syndrome that affects many Johns that goes back to a toxic escort who does us dirty. I'm lonely. I'm just like everyone else who craves love and affection. When I talk about it, people act like it's a foreign fuckin' concept. Dallas Austin gets it–that's why he wrote it in "Fanmail." And I thank him because I always feel validated because TLC put our feelings on wax.

It's why we go to sex stores when we can't afford or don't want to deal with an escort's bullshit. We get to be around other people who we can identify with in hopes of meeting with someone to take our minds away. A quick bait session or some head or the tip of someone's dick in mouth–can someone please hook me up.

Dealing with The Apprentice makes me wish I had a regular boyfriend and ironically, it's because of him that I eventually feel like this may be an option for me. I've had them before, but it's been so long since I've had anyone committed to me. I know that finding the right one for me may take longer and will be harder, but once I get him, I know and trust our communication will be better than what I'm experiencing now.

I want that for myself.

POUND CAKE

Stats
Height: 6'8"
Weight: 195 lbs
Dick Size: 9 inches

Approx. Dates or Time Frames of Encounter: 2015
Number of Encounters: 2

Cost of Encounter: $150/encounter
Performance Level: 8/10
Is the Escort Safe: Yes
ADA Friendly: Yes
Would I Recommend to Others: Yes

Card Bio: Before becoming a well-known adult entertainer who appealed to the "Blatino" crowd, Pound Cake was also well-known for his exotic dancing. Remembered for a fat, bubble-shaped ass and a spectacular muscular body to match. Every time he is seen, it's tempting to take a bite out of him. I've had the cake, eaten it and no, I'm not sharing my piece with you.

The Story:

Sometimes, I think we forget that we are in a relationship with ourselves. We have to feed, nurture and care for ourselves like newborns everyday or else are not going to be happy with the results and consequences we experience in our lives. Sex fulfills the physiological needs category of Maslow's Hierarchy and I think that's why we do and say whatever to get it. As a man, sex allows me to be dominant even as a bottom. I like being able to control my sphincter muscles to decide what kind of grip I'm going to give my top. I like that I'm able to move around and control my body movements for other people's pleasure as well as my own. As a John, I pick and control who I have a relationship with. If I don't want you, I'm not gonna reach out to you or a sexual transaction. Granted, I understand that a trick can choose not to have a relationship with me but when money is your motivator to interact with me, I do have an upper hand.

As I say this, I have to be careful when choosing a trick. I have to also be mindful and mature enough to say "no" to someone whose mental well-being may not be in a place to give me what I want. Adult performers put on the mirage that they are totally okay with grinding their nude or near nude bodies in front of a large studio audience, but we all know that many of them would choose other pathways if they thought they were obtainable. I'm mature enough now to state that some of the men whom I've had interactions with, would have been better off as therapy clients. Some would have benefited from non-sexual, almost platonic relationships with me. They should have been paying me as a confidant, and I should have in some regards, made myself more accessible to them in that way and built trust in them that they would respect me more than just the John to try to get over on.

But we are here. And as I get this off my chest by no means am I saying that Pound Cake has any of these problems. Admittedly, he is one that I wish I had met under different and better circumstances.

When I met Pound Cake, he was not in the most stable condition. His living condition was not permanent as he bounced from couch to couch, shelter to shelter. Like some of the well-known performers, Pound Cake had a history of dealing with law enforcement. According to some public records, he would be guilty of larceny and committing fraudulent activities using other people's financial resources.

If I went by watching recordings of his dancing at different adult entertainment venues, or watching his very engaging scenes on DawgpoundUSA, I wouldn't have assumed that Pound Cake had a less than perfect life.

I met Pound Cake in 2015 while dealing with and engaging with The Apprentice and trying to reconcile my relationship with Full Disclosure. We had talked, and for the most part, our conversations were friendly. We'd agree, and agreed to disagree on a lot of things going on in our community. He'd try to hold me accountable for some of the beefs I was getting into with these socialites, but be a listening ear when I needed to vent.

I'm not going to share some of the things that he told me because I do respect his privacy. And with that I didn't initially want to pursue him as a trick. The friendship I wanted with him wasn't obtainable mostly by his choice.

Knock, knock. The loud banging on the wall was disruptive to the other patrons who were staying at the Extended Stay suite I'd rented for my time in Atlanta.

I increased the speed of the motor in my wheelchair for fear he'd start kicking my door next. I opened the door and I could tell by the way he wiped the sweat from his eyes and the way his clothes gave off the scent of weed and sweat that he'd had a time getting here. He most likely ran and walked a few miles from the shelter he was staying in at the moment to the room.

"I need to take a shower," he huffed and puffed as he entered my room. Most people would be surprised to find that his voice is rather deep and not the falsetto pitch that can be heard in the bloopers outtakes on the porn videos.

I rolled my chair back from the entrance. "Go ahead. There's an extra set of towels and I have a bottle of liquid soap you can use." I offered as I watched him strip as he had it to the bathroom. If you have seen his body, you know that he was built like a solid Greek statue. The bubble of his ass was so perfect and had the right amount of muscle and fluid in it that it was hypnotizing. to top him and see what he could do with my eight and a half inches. But he'd only agree to the encounter if he topped me.

Pound Cake left the door open, inviting me to watch. He didn't close the screen door all the way and I have to admit, I wouldn't have minded him giving me a shower. While I hadn't expected it or asked, Pound Cake brought to life a version of one of my favorite videos of him. I appreciated watching him grab the bottle and squeezing a golf ball size of soap on the towel. His irises in his eyes commanded me as I helplessly grabbed my erection, freeing it from my pants.

He moved the lathered up wash cloth over his neck and across his chest, licking his lips and encouraging me to stroke. If I couldn't get a piece of that pound cake he was carrying, watching him make it was the next best thing. He continued lathering his body, making sure he cleaned each of his crevices. He grabbed some more soap and the woodsy and citrus blend amplified as his soft stick baked into a nice loaf in his hand. The way he stroked himself made me salivate, jealous that his hands were feeling that meat instead of my mouth.

He turned around and the way the wash cloth appeared and disappeared was like watching a magic trick. His ass bounced and jiggled and the next thing I know, my hands were inches from his ass. He'd previously given me consent to touch his ass prior to agreeing to this encounter.

I touched it.

I spanked it.

And it danced for me like Beyoncé in her music video.

"Take your clothes off," he invited me, reaching out from the shower, extending a hand.

It took a minute but before long, I'd joined him in the tub. I held on to the rail for dear life as he surprised me and washed my body, too. The scent from our bodies was intoxicating and the way he touched me all over was ecstasy. He gripped my chest from behind, guiding my torso down as my legs struggled to create strength it wasn't accustomed to.

"I got you," he promised as he put me at ease and penetrated me deep, easily surpassing my first and second holes. I remembered to grip him tightly as he was gentle with his strokes at first. I fantasized about working out with him and then being properly worked on in the shower. As he continued to pound me, I reached my arm back and smacked that ass twice. Even in the water, I could see that Pound Cake's ass had more bounce to the ounce.

He was who Roger & Zapp were talking about, not a Cadillac.

MILITANT

Stats
Height: 6'1"
Weight: 190 lbs
Dick Size: 10 inches

Approx. Dates or Time Frames of Encounter:
Number of Encounters: 2

Cost of Encounter: $200/hour
Performance Level: 8.5/10
Is the Escort Safe: Yes
ADA Friendly: Yes
Would I Recommend to Others: With Reservation

Card Bio: Not much is known about Militant outside of his work with DawgpoundUSA, Taggaz and other masculine presenting adult sites. What is known is that his chocolate colored skin and pretty dick to match have been known to keep fans on the edge of their seats as he pounds his partners into oblivion. According to Rent.com, he was an escort at one time or another—it's not known if he currently does this work now. Either way, no one can deny his good looks and skills he demonstrates in the bedroom

The Story:

Whoever said the best way to forget about a man was to get under a new one had a clue as to what they were talking about. I saw Militant's videos online and was attracted to the military theme he and another performer kept going in all of their videos. Even years after we were recovering from "Don't Ask, Don't Tell," it was nice to imagine this performer as an active service member (another note–if you're reading this and you're a veteran, thank you for your service). I was never one for men in uniform but the way it looked on him, I could see how it became a fetish.

Militant and I have had multiple encounters. I don't even remember the first encounter–most likely it was in a hotel but it had to have been enjoyable in order for me to agree to and pay for others. I do remember the last one. I was in Atlanta for Homecoming and to take care of some issues involving my appeal. He came and visited me a few times in my room and I trusted him enough to let him take my debit card and go shopping to get him some things, get his fee and to buy a few things I needed.

He came back and I could tell something was off because he had a body odor I wasn't familiar with. The cologne that was on top of the odor clashed with his body chemistry and I tried not to get into my feelings, but I was almost positive that he went and fucked another nigga while he was out getting my stuff.

"You want to take a shower?" I offered so I could get my mind right because I didn't want to accuse him of anything.

He non verbally accepted my offer and thank God, I had a fresh set of towels delivered to the room and one of the items he went to the store to purchase was a body wash I wanted to try. I watched him undressed and thought it was cute that he had the camouflage boxer briefs that were popular at WalMart. Shit looked good on him and I thought it was hilarious that it couldn't conceal his package or hide how firm his ass was.

As he bathed, I relished in the scent of the body wash. I don't remember the brand but I do remember how minty and woody the fragrance was and how it gave me the feeling of being in a department store trying out new scents. I wasn't big on wearing colognes at this time but I did appreciate a nice fragrance. I checked my phone and saw that the appropriate amount of money was withdrawn from my account and that another escort hit me up to see if the opportunity to get paid was still on the table. As I was declining the offer through text, Militant walked out of the bathroom drying off. I loved the way the water cascaded off his body and emphasized his physique.

"You want to take a shower before we start?" He asked.

"I'm good, I took care of that while you were out." I declined. I definitely knew something was off because he should have been able to see the damp towel I used and the pile of used towels on the floor. I made it a point to spray the bathroom with bathroom cleaner, so he should have noticed traces of ammonia and powdered bathroom cleaner when he walked in. "Unless you wanna give me another one." I flirted.

I saw the look of annoyance on his face and I hated that because I knew some disrespectful shit was getting ready to leave his mouth.

The bed was made appropriately and I made sure I had two towels on the mattress. They talk about bottoms having accidents but some of your favorite "tops" have skid marks and are musty and I don't want to see or smell that shit when I go to sleep at night.

I undressed and got on the bed. I deeply inhaled to ensure that I still smelled fresh from my shower and once I got face down, ass up, Militant got on the bed. He sat up in the bed, putting his flaccid penis in my face. I reached out to grab it and it was still soft. I lowered my head and put my lips on his tip, slowly allowing his penis to invade my mouth. I rolled my tongue and swallowed and it felt like I had a water balloon in my mouth. Instead of it getting hard, I got disappointed. Militant's dick was not getting hard and the last thing I wanted or needed on this trip was an unfulfilling sexual encounter.

"Did you fuck him while you were out?" I tried to avoid the question but this confrontation was happening. I rolled away from him and didn't bother to wipe my slobber from his dick.

"What do you mean?" He tried to play dumb.

Only pissed me off more. "Look man, I get it if I don't make you hard or whatever, but at least respect me and my time and not fuck nobody else without me when you are on my time."

Militant got up from the bed. "I told you I wasn't fuckin' no other niggas—and even if I was, I don't owe you an explanation."

"Respectfully, I wouldn't have a problem with it if I was some nigga you was getting your nut off in. But I just paid you $200 plus a tip and another $50 to go shopping for me. I waited for you for two hours in which I made sure I was properly cleaned out and that my body was fresh so you could perform. If you wanted to fuck another nigga while you was on my time, you should have at least seen if I wanted to get fucked by another nigga, too. I like trains and shit."

Militant shook his head. I knew I hit a nerve but the truth was, I didn't give a fuck. He disrespected me and he was going to have to make it up to me somehow.

"Look, I don't expect you to tell me who it is—I want to know what we gonna do about the service I paid for because I don't want a half-ass, limp dick fuck. I want what I got in our last few sessions."

"That's fair," he admitted. I had to appreciate the fact that while he pissed me off by playing off our encounter, he at least thought enough of me to try to do the right thing. "Could I come back tomorrow?"

"If you do that, then you need to leave the $200 here."

"You know I don't do refunds."

"And I don't do broken promises." I raised my voice. "I've seen this movie before and I'm still waiting for Nautica to come back from the last time."

"Nautica?" I got his attention. I should've known that Militant might have known "Nautica". I wasn't gonna mention this motherfucker because "Nautica" was another nigga that scammed me out of some money. He was supposed to send me some a private video and fuck me. I paid his fee in advance because he told me that he would make the video in my room before I got the service. At the time, I thought the idea was cool and thought it would be nice to see my video being made live and in person. Nautica came to my room with alcohol reeking from his pores. He had a bottle of cheap gin that he probably got from Kroger and stumbled into my room. I tolerated this bullshit and tried to go through with the encounter, only to find that when he stripped down to his boxers, he still had another motherfucker's scat on his dick. It was either that or he jacked his dick with some tissue he wiped his ass with. Either way, this shit was nasty and even I had standards for what I would and wouldn't do to fuck a man. Nautica promised to make it up to me and he hasn't yet.

"Yeah—you know if he around—or is he the dude you fucked?"

"You know I don't keep up with no nigga—but damn, I would've told you not to fuck with Nautica's ass. When he's not drinking, he's in the streets high as a kite." Militant confirmed.

That was disappointing to hear. I knew then I wasn't getting my money back. Another one hundred and fifty dollars, wasted.

"Well—still doesn't answer what we are going to do about my $200 man." I got back on topic. I was going to consider letting it go if he either got my money back from Nautica or got him to do a threesome with us so we could be even.

"Can you give me an hour?" Militant offered.

"As long as I don't have to pay for it." I was hoping this was going to be a set up.

I watched as Militant got back in the bed and laid next to me. Normally, he didn't cuddle and I wouldn't call this that, but the fact that he was laying next to me was cool. Not worth $200 but definitely a form of atonement. His phone rang and he reached over to where his pants were, took out the phone and declined the call. He started playing with his dick and it started gaining the strength I knew he was capable of having. The phone rang again and he did the same thing again.

"Does he want to come over?" I asked. Yeah, I was desperate for some dick but I was also willing to work with Militant to make the experience pleasurable for him. "I'm willing to watch y'all fuck if you give me a hundred dollars back."

"This is one of my other clients, he's not gonna agree to that shit."

I'm trying but I can only do so much.

"Is he more attractive to you than me?" I got right to it because I was also trying to figure out if I wanted to salvage this situation or be completely done with his ass.

"He's white and he pays more," Militant admitted. "Okay look—while I was at the store, he hit me up and I knew he wasn't too far. I told him I was busy but he offered me $500 for fifteen minutes and he promised to send a car for me. Which he did. We linked up and his driver dropped me off a few blocks away from the hotel and I walked the rest of the way here."

Damn. Militant not only fucked another guy on my time, he made an additional five hundred dollars on top of what he paid me. Escorts 2–Johns 0. I was misrepresenting us in the worst fashion.

"So just give me the $200 back and you can get it back from him. No harm, no foul."

"I'm only going to be in town for a few more hours, I'm leaving out of here tonight to go see another client in Houston."

The melancholic Drake song came to mind. I could picture him having Johns in Houston, Atlanta and Las Vegas flying him out to do his thing. As much as I wanted to get away from The Apprentice, his words and views were slapping me in the face. He used to tell me all the time about the white boys who paid him more to be with them and as much as I didn't want to make this about race, the white boys were my biggest competitors. These motherfuckers always had more money and could do the "extra" shit I couldn't do. It was bad enough that I had to be twice as good, have twice the credentials to get half the shit they get. I now had to compete with the man in a suit for a foot. Or was it some sloppy fat motherfucker that had his paws in the money bucket. Another thing about these white boys is that they had their choice of men. Black, Latino, Asian, didn't matter who they were, they always had the money to fly them out anywhere. The Apprentice once broke off a potential appointment with me so he could be with his white boy dream and now Militant was laying here breaking my heart.

I was to get sloppy seconds behind another dude he serviced on my time and was supposed to be satisfied. Where is my man and when is he getting me out of this nightmare?

"How many people did you have lined up for the day?" Shit, if I couldn't get some dick, I'd settle for the truth—for now.

"You would've been the third." I was surprised he answered.

"Three rounds, I can respect that."

Escorts 3-Johns 0. I'm fuckin' up bad.

"You should tell that to my baby mama, she is hitting the courts up to increase my child support."

I knew this shit was coming. Militant was gonna try to use sympathy so he could keep my money. I'd be out of $200 and some good dick and I wasn't going out like that. I had to get something out of this deal. "So you need this money and you're not gonna give me what I need."

"What do you want?"

"Something."

I didn't know what to ask for. I already wasn't getting no dick, I was getting pissed and I felt like I was gonna get scammed again. Why the fuck was I always falling for this shit? Every time I tried to link up with one of these motherfuckers, it was always a gamble. It was a chance they would perform and give me money's worth but it was also a chance they'd pull a stunt like this. Some man or baby mama or kid needed my money more than I needed the service I paid for.

I went for his dick again, tried playing with it, still wouldn't get hard. This was some fuck shit and I grew angrier by the second. I couldn't afford confrontation so I just told him to leave. I knew once he walked out of the door, I'd never see him again. The irony is, "Nautica" came back three or so years later and gave me a partial service for the money I'd paid. He cleaned himself up, went through rehab and while he wasn't making videos anymore, he was still doing sex work. Militant never did right by me again. Instead of dogging him, I just remember the times he brought me pleasure. He can fuck but he also fucked me over.

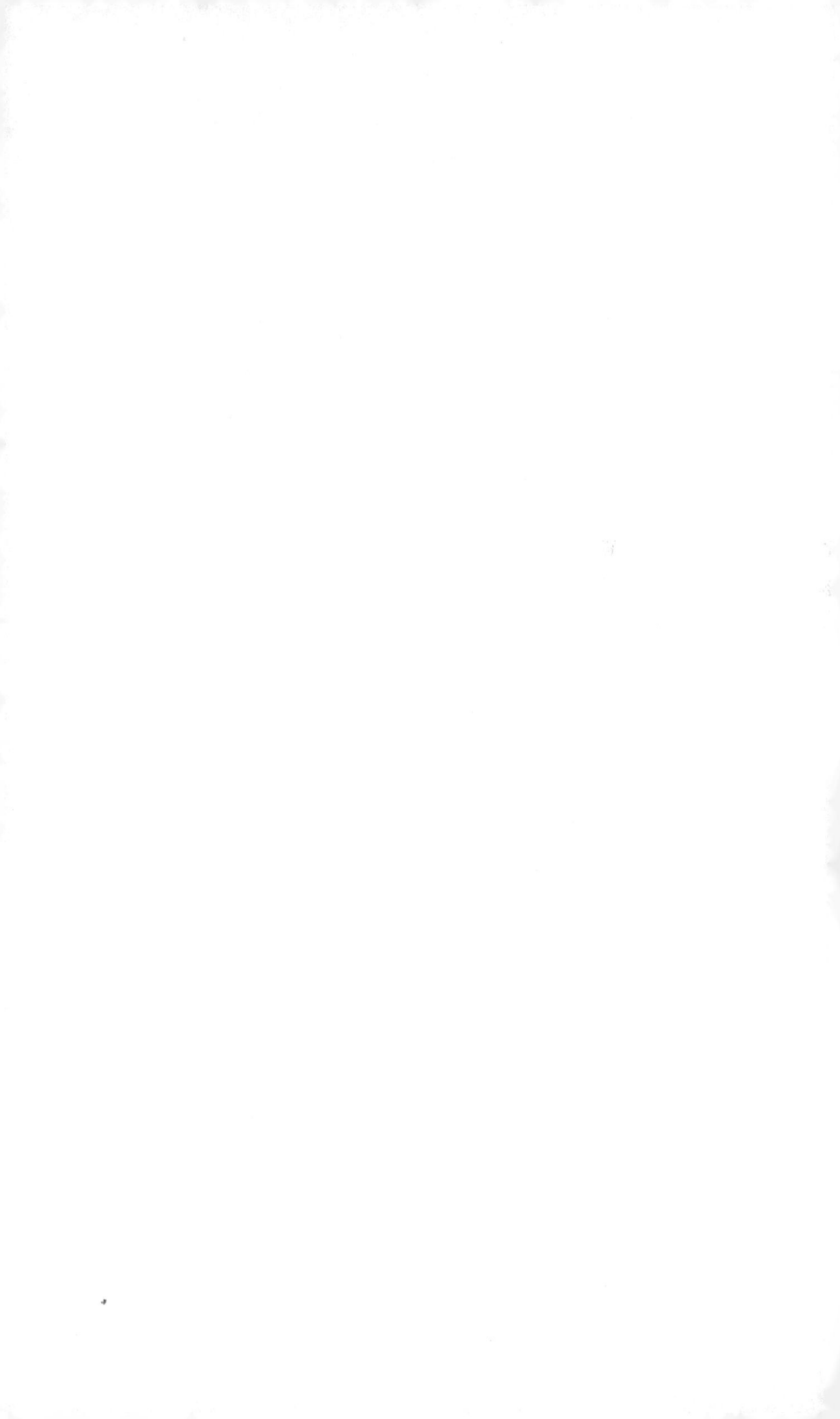

SUPHOMIE

Stats
Height: 6'1"
Weight: 180 lbs
Dick Size: 10.5 inches, uncut
Approx. Dates or Timeframes of Encounter: On Again/Off Again Since 2016
Number of Encounters: 5
Cost of Encounter: Varies based on service
Performance Level: 9.5
Is the Escort Safe: Yes
ADA Friendly: Yes
Would I Recommend to Others: Yes

Card Bio: SupHomie came to prominence in the mid-2010's in a series of videos filmed with adult studios like DawgPoundUSA, Noir Male and Treasure Island that were frequently downloaded or shared on platforms like MyVidster, Pornhub, xHamster. His thick, uncircumcised dick conceals his meaty mushroom head on soft and hangs like a banana from the tree and has a deep curve to the left. Many of his fans believe he's from Oakland or the surrounding Bay Area, given his Left Coast mannerisms and distinctive accent. He's known for filming professionally with many of the studios out there and being local to the area. SupHomie is often put into scenes where he is presented as a rough, aggressive, thugged-out top.

The Story:

After a long day of classes and some slight drama, I opened my iPhone X and noticed I missed an alert from SupHomie. I smiled because I knew he'd come through with another personalized video. I paid $150 for the last one and wondered what he would do in this one.

One of the reasons I paid for SupHomie's personal videos is because he knows how to be a good cameraman. He doesn't just put his phone on the ring light or set a camera up, press play, lay on a bed and start stroking his meat and talking shit. SupHomie gives close ups that make you think you are in the room with him. His attention to detail is immaculate because in the videos he's done for me, he's never worn the same outfit twice. It's not the same script where he pretends to come into a room, ask how my day went, and the whole "I've been missing you all day, and I hate that I can't be there" routine. SupHomie has come in off the court playing basketball; undressed to get into the shower to play in the bathroom; filmed in the car while parking in some fast food joint.

He's even, with the consent of one of another party, filmed him fucking someone live for me to view personally with no one on the stream but me.

I appreciate him for that. Most importantly, SupHomie is a real human being. We have our issues, but I like the fact that I can pick up the phone and call him, sometimes. He's not annoyed when I send him a text or an email. When we disagree, he rarely hits below the belt and when he does, he apologizes.

To an extent, SupHomie represents an ultimate goal I have for the escorts I deal with. I realize I will never be boyfriend, partner or husband to most of these dudes, but I am a human. He knows how to deal with my frailties without judgment. I've never been in his presence and felt like he was repulsed by me or my appearance. Like Aye Papi, he does wheel me around, takes care when he places me in or takes me out of my chair and from time to time, helps me out with reasonable accommodations that come with my disability. I do appreciate all of this which is why I do get disappointed when we argue and fight and go long periods of time without speaking.

If I wasn't paying him for sex, we'd probably have the makings for a good, honest friendship.

I wouldn't say we don't have that now. The truth is, I wish I'd met SupHomie under different circumstances. Perhaps I found out he was a porn star after I met him, after we became friends–maybe possibly a boyfriend. If work and things were different on my end, it might be cool for me to go to the west coast. I'd be that loving boyfriend that would suck his and his co-stars' dicks on set, manage his affairs and support his adult entertainment career no matter wherever it took him. Book his flights, tolerate the side nigga–no really, I wouldn't want him to have another man or woman besides me but if it came down to it, I'd do it.

Aye Papi is probably the only other escort that could get that from me.

I wish SupHomie was in my presence now, bending me over and plowing into me like he does the other guys in the videos I watch. The first-hand experience was way better than any video–he feels good on the inside and has good stamina. Fucks better than now than guys currently in their twenties. SupHomie gave it to me nice and rough and seeing his fitted cap meet the crease in his forehead excited me. In the background, I could see he was sitting on a navy blue towel that draped over a plush dark gray sofa. His flaccid penis appeared to be taking a nap on his thigh, his heavy balls inhaling and exhaling in a consistent rhythm.

Reminded me of the first time we had sex.

"Not bad shorty," he complimented me as he stepped into the room. I had just turned my wheelchair around so I could get into the routine of rolling to the bed and getting myself to the mattress. I was surprised when I could feel his hands on the wheelchair handles and him trying to push me forward.

"My chair is electronic," I appreciated the gesture. Not many guys offer to help me become mobile. I showed him the joystick on the right side of my chair. He cracked a smile, putting his perfect teeth on display. He leaned down and started playing with my joystick like it was part of a gaming system. Had to admire the "big kid" personality. I didn't get offended and oddly, I felt safe knowing that in our time together, SupHomie was going to take care of me.

"I can't wait to see how you move on my dick."

I wish I had filmed this encounter but to be honest, not many escorts allow me to show my full range of motion in the bedroom. Face down, ass up, drill, drill, drill. Maybe they'll cum, maybe they won't.

The hazy Teyana Taylor song played in the background of the video as SupHomie slowly pulled the hood of his hard, uncircumcised dick back in the video. Reminded that the song played in the background the first time he fucked me. This video was off to a great start and almost made me feel like a virgin again. He picked up the unlabeled jar of petroleum jelly, dug some out and put some more on his dick. I liked the way it made it look shiny. The precum started to ooze and he stopped for a moment and swiped the tip with his index finger.

"I wish this was in your mouth," SupHomie stole my thought as he played with it between his index finger and his thumb. The string was surprisingly nice and thick for it to have been such a small amount.

"I do, too." I spoke to the phone as I tossed it into my lap and wheeled myself to my bed as fast as I could. Once I got to the edge of the bed, I quickly took off my 'nalia and threw it into the dirty clothes basket. I admired my lean and well-kept upper torso and briefly thought about what I'd look like with a letter branded on my pec, but my throbbing asshole reminded me why I was kicking off my shoes so fast. I realized my milk chocolate colored dildo was in the drawer and while it wasn't SupHomie, it was gonna have to get me there. I lifted myself up from the chair, reached over to the other side of the mattress and pulled myself onto the bed. I rushed to get my pants off and hummed the chorus of Tweet's "Oops, Oh My" as I grabbed the petroleum jelly off the dresser and lather. I really needed some lube but I didn't have time or the money to go to the store to get it. I wasn't about to spit on the silicone, as I don't like the way that combination felt inside of me. I made sure to move the chuck that I had in the bed closer to the center and then position the sex toy on it. Had to make sure the balls were aiming for the foot of the bed so it would feel like I was riding him.

"You like that?" SupHomie entered my wet opening again as I felt my cheeks swallow him whole. I was still breathing hard as he had just busted a load inside me and not even five minutes of rest later, he had me on my left side, entering me again for a round two. I hoped he wouldn't charge me extra for this but I just paid him $400 for two hours of his time.

"Yes." I moaned as the stubble from pubic hairs brushed the hair on my ass. I like the fact that he was freshly shaven. Even with my right leg in the air and SupHomie breathing down my back, I still loved the way his heavy balls managed to slap mine. The strokes were hitting deeper as my hole tightened and got wetter.

SupHomie had just worked me while I laid on my back. I could feel the sweat from his chest dab my shoulder. My nipples felt like they were on fire from the way he was twisting them earlier. I moaned and screamed his real name as he filled me up again. Not long after, my dick got thicker as I wet the bed.

I'd never pissed before while getting fucked and I was so ashamed. I looked down and was glad that I had a towel and a chuck on the bed, but even with that, I knew I was going to have to have the motel bring me some new sheets.

"*Damn, you soaker for real?*" SupHomie chuckled as he laid in the bed with me. *It was a nice change not to see the escort quickly jump up as they tell you a few things as you see them from the back as they are off to quickly get away from you.*

"*This has never happened before.*" I was ashamed because the last thing I wanted was for him to think I pissed in the bed on purpose. I was thirty - four years old and way too old for this shit.

"*I'm hitting that spot if I'm making you piss the bed man. I don't mind that shit.*" SupHomie stretched out and put his hands behind his head. "*Just don't piss on me when you're riding.*"

Duly noted.

On cue, the silicone penis head penetrated my hole as SupHomie encouraged me to stroke my dick while I was riding him. The phone had fallen to the side and I quickly picked it up so that I could see him stroking his wet dick as I felt my meat fatten in my left hand. I bounced up and down on the silicone, listening to SupHomie grunt and take me down memory lane to when he had fucked me before. In the first video, he reminded me that I deserved to enjoy sex and be treated with respect. I missed the man scent from his pubes as I longed for another dildo to use while I dreamed of sucking his dick. I loved the way his real dick pulsating in my mouth. I squeezed my nipple as he had many times before and I started riding the dildo faster. I could feel my dick stiffen and my nut churning at the bottom of my balls. I imagined his grip on my dick tightening as I was about to cum.

"Get that nut niggah!" He encouraged me as I felt myself getting there.

The sweat from my cheeks tricked me into thinking his hands were caressing my thighs and cupping my ass. I rode the dildo harder and faster. He encouraged me to cum and before long, that's exactly what I'd done.

"You's a nasty bitch!" SupHomie laughed as I licked my cum off his belly button and pretended to suck on it like I was sucking his dick. I looked in his eyes and smiled wickedly as I wiped his lubed and asscreamed dick with my bare hands.

"Oh, I can get nasty." I hated when he challenged me but just to show him I wasn't one to be fucked with, I moved between his legs and grabbed his dick and swallowed him whole. No practice, no hands, I had all of him in my mouth in one shot. I went up and down as he patted my head and then grabbed my growing locks. The feeling of my hair follicles expanding as he continued to move my head up and down excited me. I knew he could smell my freshly fucked ass as I did as I breathed in and out on his pubes. He held me in place as I could feel his moment come, too. I got back up to the tip of his dick. I moved his foreskin up and down real fast and when I felt his vein expand, I quickly put his dick back in my mouth. I was going back to Cali and he was going to the back of my throat and into my stomach as he gave me a fresh shot of protein. I sucked and sucked as I felt his fingers tickle my ass.

This was beyond wonderful, I was in heaven.

The bliss brought me back to reality as he was encouraging me to calm down. SupHomie knew me so well that he knew when I was gonna cum and probably figured out what I was going to do to get off. I wanted to fuck him again but he was already booked for his upcoming trip to Atlanta. It would be almost a year before he folded me up again. My ass throbbed and I moved the cursor on my phone to the beginning of the video. I marked the video as a favorite as I made my way back onto the dildo and began the process all over again.

SOMEDAY IS TONIGHT

So now comes the question, was it worth it? Meeting with the escorts, the thrilling link ups. Getting robbed or physically hurt. Doing almost anything to meet one of my Maslow's hierarchy of needs.

On the outside looking in, I could see why you'd be like why are we fucking with these niggas?

I admit it is a valid question. Why am I fucking with these niggas? They are the other side of this equation. In addressing what they want, their needs appear to be simple, money.

They want money.

And there's nothing wrong with being a sex worker and making an honest living, providing a service there means if we're being honest. Before you judge me or even judge them, ask yourself, do you have a boyfriend? Do you have a person or two that you can rely on to fulfill your sexual needs at the spur of the moment? Who are they, and what are they to you? Meshell Ndegeocello could not have asked the question better herself.

I do acknowledge the risk that the sex workers put themselves in when they attempt to meet people like me. Yes, you see me in my chair. It's known that I have a physical disability. I've paid my deposit, and oftentimes, paid for your plane ticket, train ticket, or some other ride to my location. Yeah, even though I fulfill my end of the bargain when initiating these transactions, I do acknowledge that not everyone does the same. I do know and acknowledge that sex workers walk into unfamiliar territory, only to be attacked, robbed, or have other things that could happen to jeopardize their lifestyles. I do know and understand that giving eight to thirteen inches a pleasure two to three times a day for seven days a week does create an irreparable rip on the bodies, mind, consciousness, and soul.

I acknowledge all of that.

I argue that the John takes the greatest risk. Nine times out of ten, we are inviting the sex worker into our home—not a hotel, a park, or some other place where we can randomly meet up. These people come into our homes, and have immediate access to our lives. Most of us cannot afford to pay for separate apartments, condos, suites for our carnal pleasures. We'll do all of this because everyone should be able to have their sexual needs met in the environment in which they should feel the safest. By bringing these men to our home, we set ourselves up. Who's to say that the sex worker's side gig isn't robbing random motherfuckers? The sex worker is able to come into our home, learn the layout of our land, and that will take advantage of us in our most vulnerable spot.

The John is the most vulnerable in this situation, because in 2024, we have to pay a deposit to book the service. In most cases not only is the deposit non-refundable, it's hard to dispute the transaction with the credit card companies and banks if something goes wrong. Our risk is that we can set up a time place and the agreed upon deposit is submitted and the performer does not show up. Or they try to offer us a non-fulfilling alternative so they could half ass do the work we paid them to do. We are already on the losing end of this situation because we paid the deposit, yet we don't receive the service we paid for.

Where is that right?

Assuming one can take legal action and convince a judge or arbitrator to hear our case, they will mention if the transaction is illegal in their jurisdiction–if so, there's no recourse. Everyone else is like "you put yourself in this situation. Why should I feel sorry for you?"

That's not what we're asking for. We're asking you to understand that we deserve to be treated as human beings, who are capable of love and affection And deserve to be treated just as good if not better than how we treat other people.

So, in addition to paying our deposits, letting them enter our homes, one of our biggest risks is having our dream turn into a nightmare. We suffer a trauma for which few are willing to treat or give an acceptable cure. How many times have *we* rewind the sex scene? Then they come to us and their dicks can't get hard. Wait a minute. That's not what I saw in the videos. That's not what went viral on social media. I've grab limp dick after limp dick and would have done better bending the motherfucker over and fucking them with my dick. With all of my ailments and physical transgressions, I can get a hard on without relying on drugs, or videos, or supplements. When the fantasy turns into a sham, we are the ones who are disappointed. I don't wanna video chat when I pay for a sexual performance. I don't want an "exclusive" picture that you probably sent to all your private clients that anyone can post on the net instead of the performance. If I pay your fucking ass $250, $500, over $1000, I want the performance! I'm paying for your rock hard dick to make my hole throb. My body to be put through a rigorous exercise.

I want your version of Kanye's "Workout Plan." That's what I'm paying for.

Chances are if I've hit you up for a sexual performance, I've already subscribed to your subscription sites to see the videos that are not on social media. I've probably paid a couple of dollars for a private conversation. And\or tipped you in a few of your videos just so that I could be a thought in your mind.

I've done my part. The last thing I want is a shitty ass performance.

So what happens when you do get to my house and the dick doesn't get hard? Everyone wants to sing the Rick Ross mantra "money makes me cum?" But when you see the Benjamins and Jacksons on the table, or the ding chimes on your merchant app, and you still can't bring me what I need.

So I ask who is being cheated?

While I'm blessed with the ability to make multiple streams of income despite my physical disability, I know there are others that aren't as blessed as I am in that department. Some Johns have lost various portions of their mental capacity. So I have to speak up for them because no one is speaking up for us. Some of these men spend their whole disability check in hopes of having an encounter and many times they are robbed by the people you jack your dicks to. That's part of the reason some of these guys got into sex work. It's easy to rob people who are unable to defend themselves, don't have a voice, can't get an advocate, point you out in the line up.

To the upcoming sex workers, I want to warn you that your average John is not gonna look like your colleagues that you feel content with. Their is an allure to get the rich white men who have six-figure incomes or higher but in order to get to that crowd, you have to know the right person and oftentimes that's not gonna come with a ballroom membership. To attract the rich and wealthy clients that have halfway decent luxe, you have to be able to show that you can earn the money outside of sex. You have to be able to provide other services that are marketable and will get you a job anywhere. Having a college degree can help, being a member of a fraternity or respected social organization can be better, but if you don't have your own property and your own bank account, then you're not gonna meet the men you think you deserve to seek.

Who wants you in their house when you don't belong there?

And trust, these men have a way of finding us. They know if you've dealt with us. Karma has a nasty way of dealing with you when you rob and steal from your Johns. Miss treat your Johns. There's a reason why some of the sex workers who were popular in the 99's in 2000's can't even do content creation now.

Those of us who have been around the block will tell you to be careful how you treat someone. Don't assume that because you are currently in better physical shape than your typical John, that you're going to forever be able to overtake him. Quiet as his kept, many of the Johns with the physical and mental disabilities are still connected to the rich and powerful families you wish you could provide services to. The John doesn't always have to tell them that you are scamming them. The person they're paying to watch that John is going to tell it.

But this is neither here nor there. Sometimes it's worth it because as I am venting about sex workers taking advantage of people and providing horrible customer service, I do acknowledge that there are few who always do right by me. I'll know when they go I'm able to contact them I'm going to get what I paid for, and I'm going to be done right. Ironically, those people can be the hardest to get in contact with. They don't always need or want the money that comes with doing sex work because they themselves have other streams of income that sustains them.

My goal and idea when I communicate my wants and needs and desires to a sex worker is that it will be worth it in the end. I want a memorable experience that I can keep in my memory bank. I want the pleasure to be real for me. I don't want to be another piece of ass that's looked down upon because I've paid for something that I deserve to have access to for free.

The world would be perfect. If I didn't have to pay for dick, and people didn't have to sell their pussy ass dick in lips. Commerce for comfort. Wish you were there.

Allegedly, in other universes prostitution doesn't exist.

But we are on this one.

AFTERWORD

BY CEDRIC QUINCY

What I Learned About Sex From a Disabled Person's Perspective.

Prior to collaborating with Tony for *Don't Get F+cked Up* and *Piece of Ass,* I first researched about people with disabilities having sex for a novel I wrote called *King* by Cedric Quincy & Donte Sweat (yes, I write under both pseudonyms–long story). This erotic thriller was built on revenge for the murder of King's disabled younger brother. One of the frequent questions I'm asked is if the sex scenarios I wrote about King's brother experiencing were real?

To that, I answer with a resounding *yes!!!*

At the time, I worked as a direct care worker for those with special needs. My job required that I help people work on tasks needed to live a fulfilling life and help them with daily activities of living as needed. In my line of work, I met with several parents and guardians who openly discussed "sex dates" for their relatives. I know of situations where clients regularly met with "peers" and/or "sex workers" and encouraged them to "Get It On", as Marvin Gaye would say. Like many who would appear "normal", I was appalled and even felt the behavior was abusive. Then my eyes were opened when I witnessed a service provider bringing some of their clients to an adult bookstore. I watched these men and women enter the store, walk around the theater and participate in some of the same activities with other patrons.

It was that moment that made me appreciate the level of sexual freedom I had. Even if I'm not happy with my appearance or self-conscious about other things—many of the disabled unintentionally bring their physical limitations to their sexual encounters. I realized then that many of these people are repressed sexually and I remember some of my colleagues reprimanding and punishing clients for expressing themselves sexually. Granted, it was one thing to "whip it out" or put your fingers down in a public setting. It's another to reprimand them for expressing themselves in the bathroom or in their rooms.

When Tony and I discussed writing *Piece of Ass*, it was supposed to be a separate section of the autobiography. One place where Tony would have been able to deftly define his sexual identity and even talk about some of the "famous people" he's had sexual experiences with. Once I outlined the book and watched Tony interact with the personalities on different reality shows, I realized how many of those personalities thought they were above him because they were physically able or "aesthetically pleasing" and to them Tony was not. Some of these people have scammed Tony from sexual and nonsexual services that were solicited. A few of these people would not have done the things with other people who would be identified as able-bodied.

In researching celebrities and other people who discussed sex in their biographical books and films, some went into more details than others. Not to deny anyone's belief that sexual acts between two or more people should be private, but I think that a lot of people don't see folks with disabilities as sexual beings. Many people don't visit their relatives in group homes or assisted-living centers and I know this from personal experience. At best, people with physical and mental disabilities are background characters in everyone else's stories. They're mentioned as "asides" or in the form of "charity work" they do.

Listening to Tony talk in-depth about his personal experiences with prostitutes and engaging in paid sexual encounters with random people changed my own perspective. This view point is one of the reasons why I believe sex work should be legal, regulated and taxed. All people deserve to experience sex consensually and consciously. My true feelings are that sex should be free—however, if sex has a price, it should be one that all parties are willing to pay.

I'm happy that the decision was made to make *Piece of Ass* a separate book. I feel that Tony's story, and others who've shared them with me, deserve to be told. We all need a lesson in compassion. We need to learn to see *all* people as individuals that deserve to live fulfilling lives.

I hope that in telling Tony's story, people with physical disabilities get the sexual liberation they deserve.

WORKS CITED

Noir Male (MenofPorn.Net) - Various visits since June 1, 2020

"The Apprentice" Corporation - Various visits sense June 1, 2020

"Powerful concubines and influential courtesans" Published online by Cambridge University Press: 05 July 2016

https://www.cambridge.org/core/books/prostitutes-and-matrons-in-the-roman-world/powerful-concubines-and-influential-courtesans/DCC15FC6A35D368295EB82C9EE2193C4

ACKNOWLEDGMENTS

If you only know what it take to get to this moment you be surprised. I like to thank my co author and now friend of six years Cedric Quincy. All my family and friends for supporting my endeavors. Special shoutout to my friend Dre AKA IceKreamFreak for getting into my ass about my brand and letting my voice be hear and taking things seriously. Even when I wanted to give up. Also Shoutout to Freakzilla AKA Dru for creating amazing book covers and providing his wisdom with his 20 plus years career in the porn industry. Last but not least a great photographer in @Vanick on IG thank you for some of the amazing images you may see throughout the book!

Visit Me Online at www.rollonrebel.com

Follow Me on Twitter: @rollonrebel
Follow Me on Instagram: @rollonrebel

Like My Facebook Page: Rollon Rebel

Email Me: rollonrebel@gmail.com

ABOUT THE AUTHORS

Since birth, **TONY REBEL** has had to fight for his place in society. Not letting his disabilities define him, Rebel has worked to become a strong advocate for people with mental and physical disabilities and those on the LGBTQIA spectrum. A graduate of The University of Missouri-St. Louis and Webster University, Rebel works as a mental health professional. He lives with his family in Atlanta, Georgia.

CEDRIC QUINCY is a private family man that is settling down from traveling on the wild side. He stays discreet to protect his family from his shenanigans.

A Preview of the Book Y'all Heard So Much About

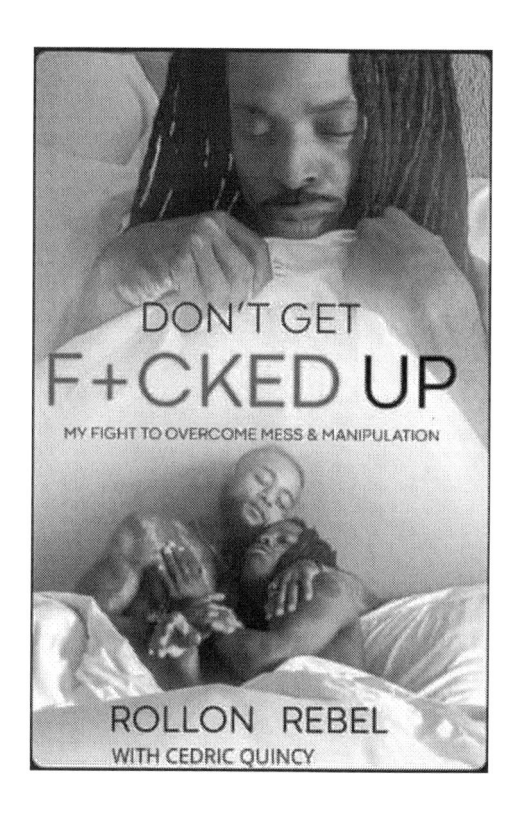

DON'T GET F+CKED UP
MY FIGHT TO OVERCOME MESS & MANIPULATION

Available in Print & eBook Formats wherever books are sold

INTRO: POST UP!!

"The next time I see you, I'm a smack the shit out of you!"

I wanted to see that promise fulfilled. This porn star/actor named Quan and I were friends at one point, or at least I thought we were friends. Quan was my friend when he wanted to borrow some money, or needed an ear to vent, or needed encouraging words to make himself feel better. He had a rough life at least in public from what we could see.

When I first saw Quan on the computer screen, it's almost as if we had a bond. He and I weren't that much different. We both are young, college-educated black men with potential. The fact that he had a physical deformity drew me closer to him, it was another trait we both had in common.

The intentions with this man were on some good-vibes shit. I saw Quan as an actor in quite a few webseries produced by independent black LGBTQ filmmakers. One could log into YouTube and see him in a variety of roles. When Quan wasn't on my computer screen trying to portray the straight-acting gay boy next door, he was modeling on

Instagram. I respected his hustle. Quan looked good with his clothes on and his clothes off and he appeared to do a good job representing us. He put his six foot, one hundred and seventy pound track star frame to work as a background dancer for a few respected independent artists.

Quan needed help because while there were fans who knew him as a YouTube actor and personality, his past was beginning to haunt him. Led by some jealous actors and nobodies, they'd dug up some private sex videos, some of which were recorded and/or shared without his knowledge or consent. His enemies on these shows not only shared these videos with their friends and fans, they ridiculed him about his past life decisions. It was so bad, it was almost to the point where they were bullying him. Like many in our small, backbiting, nosy ass community, I too, had seen the videos. The man could teach a college course on how to deepthroat a Coke bottle. And he took the kind of dick women only dreamed of. Yeah, we saw the videos.

It wasn't the first time I'd seen him on film. I saw the work he'd done for a few prominent adult video companies and when I thought we were friends, he confided in me about how he wanted to separate his adult life from his public persona. When he first stepped on the reality show circuit, he wanted to focus more on acting with his clothes on. Expand on opportunities to showcase his ability to model and dance. Be a positive influence on young black gay youth.

In our friendship, I had given the man consultation and suggested ideas on how he could do just that. We had similar goals and aspirations and I wanted to see him achieve and give his haters the middle finger.

Without being reminded that he could take dick while doing a headstand.
 I felt he could do it. I supported him and wanted to see him succeed at becoming the person he said he wanted to be. Which is why we laughed, cried and texted each other for the past year and a half. Which is why I went apeshit when one of his cast mates or a member of the audience would try to bring up his past. I was sick of him not being able to move beyond being someone's fetish. Talking about him being a porn star and trashing him in public while sliding in his DM's, begging for a piece of ass behind the scenes. Speculating about his health while wanting the same treatment he'd given another costar. The hypocrisy of it all.
 And what did I want?
 If you asked me six months ago, the answer was to be his friend and to help him realize he is a beautiful human being—with or without his clothes on. Remind him that his education wasn't in vain and if he used it wisely, he could start his own business. Unlike those who shaded him or shamed him for clout, Quan had obtained his bachelor's degree and he worked in a well-respected job that afforded him the ability to live in his own apartment. He could buy a car if he wanted to. He had a respectable nine to five and I felt that if he wanted to move up in that, he could. Truthfully, I would have taken great joy in watching him have his cake and eat it too because brothers like us don't get the spotlight. If my public defense of his words and actions cost me some potential friendships along the way, I could give two fucks because what y'all not gonna do, is try to jump on and play him.

Today, at this very moment, however, he and I have a score to settle. Somewhere between defending his right to be what he wanted to be and what he wanted to be true, Quan got it in his mind that I was an enemy. He switched up on me while I was having a war of words on his behalf with his cast mates. Told me I wasn't shit. Called me a stalker and accused me of wanting to fuck him.

All of a sudden, I was becoming acquainted with a two-facested, gutter-mouth, backstabbing bitch I couldn't stand. Words of appreciation and gratitude were replaced with "I don't know him." This motherfucker doesn't know me but slides in my DM's, wanting to talk, wanting twenty dollars for food, wanting sympathy. Mind you, between his legitimate job and his side hustles, he shouldn't need money for food or random shit that comes up. But I give all three because I thought we were becoming friends and as his friend, I wanted to see him make it. What I didn't know was he was being greasy with me.

It hurt me to know Quan was using me. I had been finessed by someone who used pity parties to find his next victims. The fact that people who knew him came back to me with the information--bragging about getting over on me. Y'all better watch his ass.

The hurt and betrayal led me here. The words and insults that were frequently hurled at one another brought me over five hundred miles to come face to face for the first time. Not that we hadn't FaceTime before—but physical presence.

For the past few weeks, Quan has called me out of my name, made accusations about my character and threatened violence against me.

He was gonna slap the shit out of me.

He was gonna roll me and my chair down the flight of stairs.

He was gonna do this—he was gonna do that.

Well, show me damnit. I want all the smoke you think I got coming my way. Fuck all this talking shit. And fuck everything about you.

With all the arguing and commotion going on at the Level Up Reunion that was being filmed at an event center in Buckhead, I rolled my ass up to him the first chance I got. I was ready to see those hands. I wanted to see if he could tip me out of the chair—but I was gonna knock the shit out of him first. See, what people got fucked up is they think just because I'm in this damn chair that I'm a pushover. Motherfuckers think they can talk about me any kind of way. And that I'm gonna sit there and take it.

There he was in the flesh—-wearing a mesh colored shirt and some ripped black jeans. The woody and citrus undertones of the cologne he wore penetrated my nose and caused a sudden dislike for the scent. I was ready.

"Ayo, Quan!" I called his name and he looked a little frightened when he saw me. Even though he told production I could come and that he'd be ready for me, I could see he was all bark and no bite. The thing next to fear is to pretend nonexistence but this motherfucker saw me. Quan knew who I was.

Before I could reach out and touch him better than Diana Ross ever could, I was being rolled away. One of the security guard's production had moved me out of the way as they were having their hands full with the other conflicts. Seems like I wasn't the only one with a score to settle. Their security was a step up from the previous season. I looked for him, expecting him to sneak a blow from behind or to be tussling with security to give me those hands.

When our eyes met, I heard part of the conversation where he was asked about me.

"I don't know him." Quan lied as he looked me in the eyes.

The screenshots in my phone say differently. Whatever. I see his punk ass for all that he is and now I know for myself that he doesn't have my respect. If you're gonna talk shit about me, back it up. Don't say you're gonna do this—gonna do that—and when I show up to the spot, don't deliver. Cause I promise you, you'll get fucked up messing with me.

I'm tired of these people taking my kindness for weakness. Thinking because I'm in this chair they can walk all over me. What they don't know is that I've been fighting all my life. For my life. Always having to prove myself to someone. Show people that I can do it.

It's all good. Like Ice Cube said, "I see the bitch in you," and from now on, I don't know you either. As I was being wheeled to a pickup location on the property, I debated whether I was gonna give this motherfucker any more shine. But I'm good. He's not the only reason I came back to the A. I have scores to settle—and I didn't know it, but I'd get into some more shit before this trip was over with. Right now, other than figuring out where I'm gonna go next, I'm sorting out where I'm going to take the journey from here.

The thing is people think they know me and they only know bits and pieces of me. They ask all kinds of questions and make speculations about what they think they see in me. I'm tired of that shit, too. I'll tell my own story—let me start at the beginning.

1. I STARTED OUT A SECRET...

According to my mother, she did not know that my father was married or that he had a family. In 1980, when the affair started, the internet had not been made public. Black Entertainment Television, otherwise known as BET, had been founded but spent its small window of broadcast time running reruns and music videos by black artists. The radio stations played pop music, country and discussed community events—not gossip. Local scandals didn't make it to the classified sections of the major newspapers and *Ebony, Jet, RightOn!* and other magazines wouldn't have covered it because my parents weren't celebrities. From what I know, my mother didn't run in the circles that my father and his family were in and any co-worker on the bus line who knew my father was married didn't feel it was any of their business to share the news with her.

What I do know is that his vision of the future did not include me.

On November 17, 1981, I became the youngest of five siblings with a brother and sister from each of my parents. I was born with cerebral palsy. It's a neurological disease that affects the body and the brain. Depending on the person it can affect you differently. It doesn't affect me that bad. It affects me in a sense of being able to walk normally like everybody else. I can go about my everyday life. It's just known that I have this disability however because I have cerebral palsy, I, like everyone else, will lose function of my body parts if I don't use them. I am at that age where that can take place so I am constantly working to be active so these things don't happen.

By all accounts, I've always had a good upper body dexterity—I'm very good at moving my hands and arms. I can do a push up on the floor or a pull up if the bar is low enough for me to reach from my chair. When I was younger, I had better standing ability—but lower body dexterity was where I struggled the most. I could stand and walk a very limited distance. I usually moved to and from class, down the hallway. My abilities faded more in middle school after I started puberty. When I got older in middle school and high school, I became very dependent on a wheelchair. I had a walker, but struggled with it—especially when I had to walk longer distances. After a while, I stopped trying.

Now, I primarily get around via my electric wheelchair. When I'm in a car or some place that does not have a ramp, I do have a manual wheelchair I can use if I have to. Being in the wheelchair doesn't mean that I'm not independent. I can take a bath and clean myself thoroughly—I don't need assistance when going to the bathroom. Obviously, I can't stand and take a piss without rails to hold or a wall to lean on, but I'm capable of getting to the bathroom and relieving myself on the toilet, provided my access isn't blocked. Yes, I prefer the handicapped stalls because I use the rails to help me get to the toilet from the chair. I'm able to wiggle my toes, move my legs, I can stand for short periods of time. When I'm in bed, I can turn freely.

In all honesty, part of this was my fault because if I worked a little harder, I probably could stand better and walk longer distances with a walker. The truth is, I became dependent upon the chair. Not that I wanted a servant or an aide to push me around and do things for me—but I'd get discouraged when my legs would give out or I didn't make a therapeutic goal I wanted to achieve. I gave up and that's where I fucked up. I admit to wallowing in the laziness but I knew I had to get to where I needed to get to. When I was in high school and transitioning from different classes, I only had a certain amount of time to get there. They made accommodations for me for certain things, it just became easier for me to move around in the chair. It became a normal way of life and I got used to it. The other half of that is just that it is what it is. Things change.

Back to my family, my mom worked as a bus operator for thirty-two years. I love my mom, but like many single parents, she worked her ass off to take care of her three children, so she was not always around because she was working. Dee Dee, my sister, who was fourteen at the time I was born, stepped up and became my primary caretaker in my youth. Darron, my older brother, was thirteen when I came around. With that being said, there is a partial generation gap between them and me. They were born in the late sixties/early seventies, I came along in the early eighties. Between that, and the power dynamic with Dee Dee being like my mother and some confusion with who's role was whose. So it's easy to understand why there's a lot of resentment with my mom even though I don't even though they don't talk about it. And even now, everything has to be run by them.

They are always trying to protect me. They see me as the little boy that they always want to protect and shield.

Darrrn was the wild middle child who was jealous because he felt like I was a perfect child, the college educated one. "You think you know everything. You think you better than me." He'd scold and tease me.

The other part of the reason was that Darron would go on to abuse drugs. He did his thing and I just watched him. So I felt like I had to take on the role of big little brother. And that's where our relationship has always been. It's like, I can't stand you, I hate you because everything you do affects me. Now my mom feels like she has to be more watchful in taking care of me because of the shit you've done.

It's kinda hard to explain. I've always resented Darron because he always made me question who I was and made fun of me. And never encouraged me to be me. It's hard to talk about. We have gotten closer because of the turn of events. My brother's health has declined. He's had strokes, diabetes and congestive heart failure. This was brought on by all the years of drug abuse. Our relationship has changed but I don't know if it is safe to say that we're close because there is still some hurt and pain there.

When Darron and I weren't at each other's throats, we were really good friends. He'd do some of the therapy work with me, but he'd spoil me too by picking me up instead of encouraging me to use my walker or he'd bring me food from one of the fast food restaurants he worked at.

At my elementary school, I decided to participate in the talent show in the fourth grade. He bought me a St. Louis Cardinals hat and jersey and dressed me backwards so I could look like Kris Kross and recite the words to their hit, "Jump."

My mom and my sister couldn't come because they were working, so I enjoyed seeing Darron in the front row, cheering me on.

If I had to compare the relationship with my brother to the one with my father, I'd say my brother was the best thing since sliced bread, while my father viewed me as the piece of mold he'd scrape off the piece of bread he had to eat so he wouldn't waste it.

My father was barely in my life—I knew him and I knew he didn't love or care about me. I didn't understand that my mom was the side piece or that she was allowing him to use her for just sex. When he came over, he rarely acknowledged my presence—all he wanted was whatever she was willing to give him. I'm not going to say my mother didn't try to encourage my father to have a relationship with me. She did suggest that he could still play catch with me, he could roll with me down the block and just talk and shoot the shit. Do things fathers are supposed to do with their children. But he never did any of that—he wanted nothing to do with me. My mom would piss me off because she was still sleeping with him and rewarding his neglectful behavior toward me.

I may have been nine or ten when I had a decent conversation with the man. That may have been the last time the two of them were intimate. I knew they worked at the same company and it's possible that their relationship started while they drove busses—but I never saw the two of them together for any concert, family gathering or important milestone I had.

It was bad enough that I was the secret child, but worse that I was a handicapped child. My father couldn't be bothered with that.

The fucked up thing is that my father had time for my brother—the one my mother had by someone else. He'd take him places and do things with him. Dee Dee would bite her tongue and try not to curse him out when she saw him—Darron would play it cool. Sometimes, he'd give me the gifts from my father—sometimes he wouldn't. Once he'd been able to get on the bus or ride in the passenger's side of his friend's rides, he'd hardly make time for my old man.

Can't blame him—Darron didn't have a relationship with his or Dee Dee's father.

This is how my life started. My mother, God bless her soul, worked day and night driving the bus all over St. Louis. Dee Dee was my second mother and head of the household because not only did she look after me, but she managed being my caretaker while raising her own kids.

You know how at the beginning of the chapter I told you I had a brother and sister from each parent? Well, I've never met my brother and sister from my father. My mother would tell me as we were editing this book that she didn't find out about his children until I was in my twenties. My father never told me I had other siblings so I don't know their names, if they have children—which I imagine to be the case because they are at least five years older than Dee Dee. I don't hold any ill will toward them because who knows if they know about me. But if there is a chance for a connection, I'd welcome it with open arms.

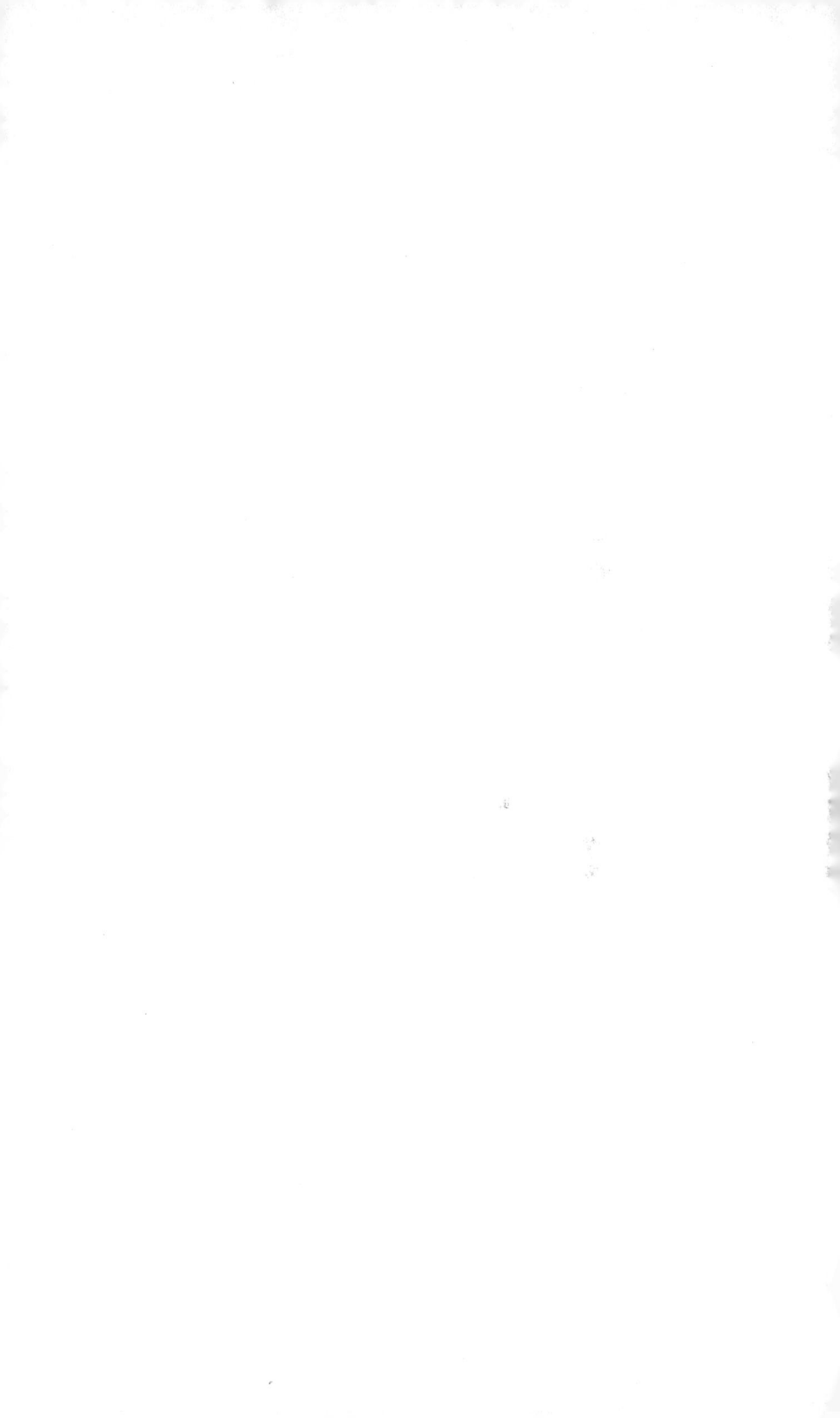

Made in the USA
Columbia, SC
18 August 2024